# MANDALA

## Coloring Book For
## Adult Art Therapy Anti Stress

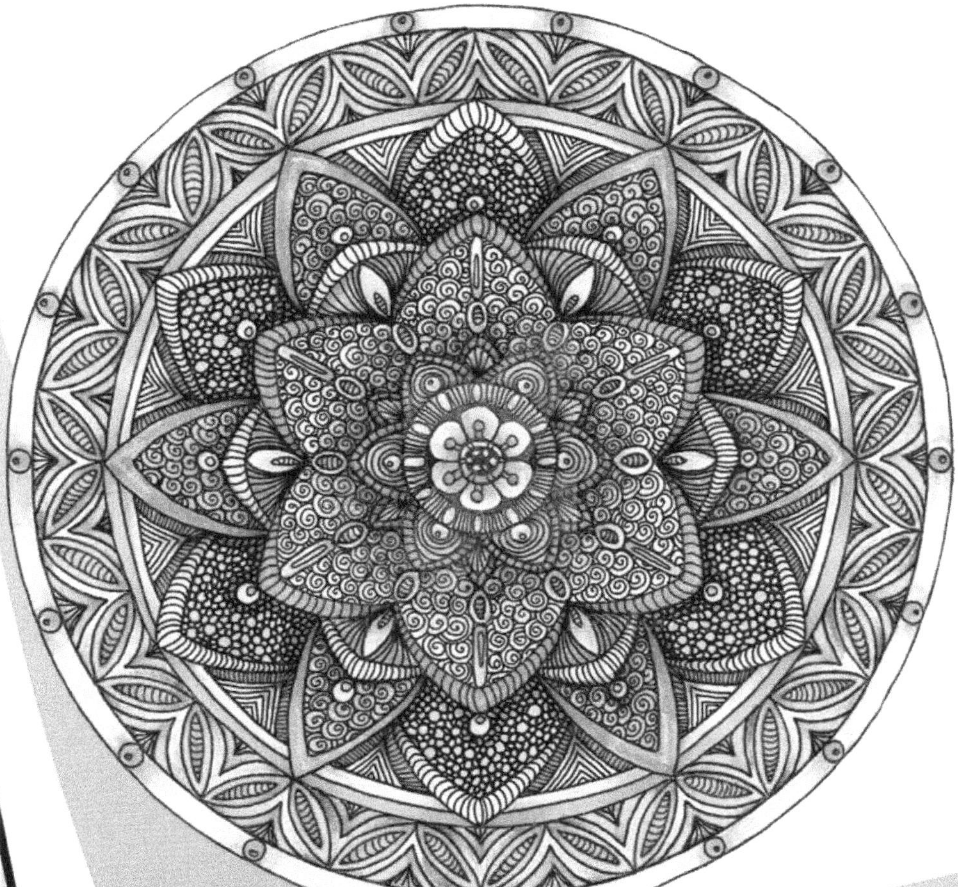

LENKA SARKHELOVA

# Copyright © 2018  by Lenka Sarkhelova



**First Printing, 2018**

**ISBN- 9781728912516**

# INTRODUCTION

Are you looking for a relaxing hobby that is easy to follow and doesn't require any huge financial investments? Would you like to reconnect with your childhood memories and have a fun time, or you're simply searching for an original gift idea that would make the day for a special friend? Do you like to draw or color? The Mandala Animals coloring book is the ideal solution!

With over 80 pages of unique animal designs, this adult coloring book is one of the largest on the market, keeping you entertained and engaged for hours! Whether you're just starting to discover this lovely hobby or you're already at advanced stages, this book is definitely a must in your collection. Its superior quality paper and versatile models allow you to use any coloring tools you like, from markers, gel pens, Crayola or even watercolors. You'll feel more relaxed and stress-free while developing and letting loose your creative spirit and imagination!

**7 benefits of coloring books for adults:**

- Stress and anxiety can be lowered
- Your mind will enter a meditative state
- You will think more positively and negativity will be expelled
- You will become more creative and happy
- You can take this coloring hobby with you wherever you go
- It can be enjoyed by anyone
- It is not an expensive hobby

Order now and invest in this activity that will keep your mind healthy and happy!

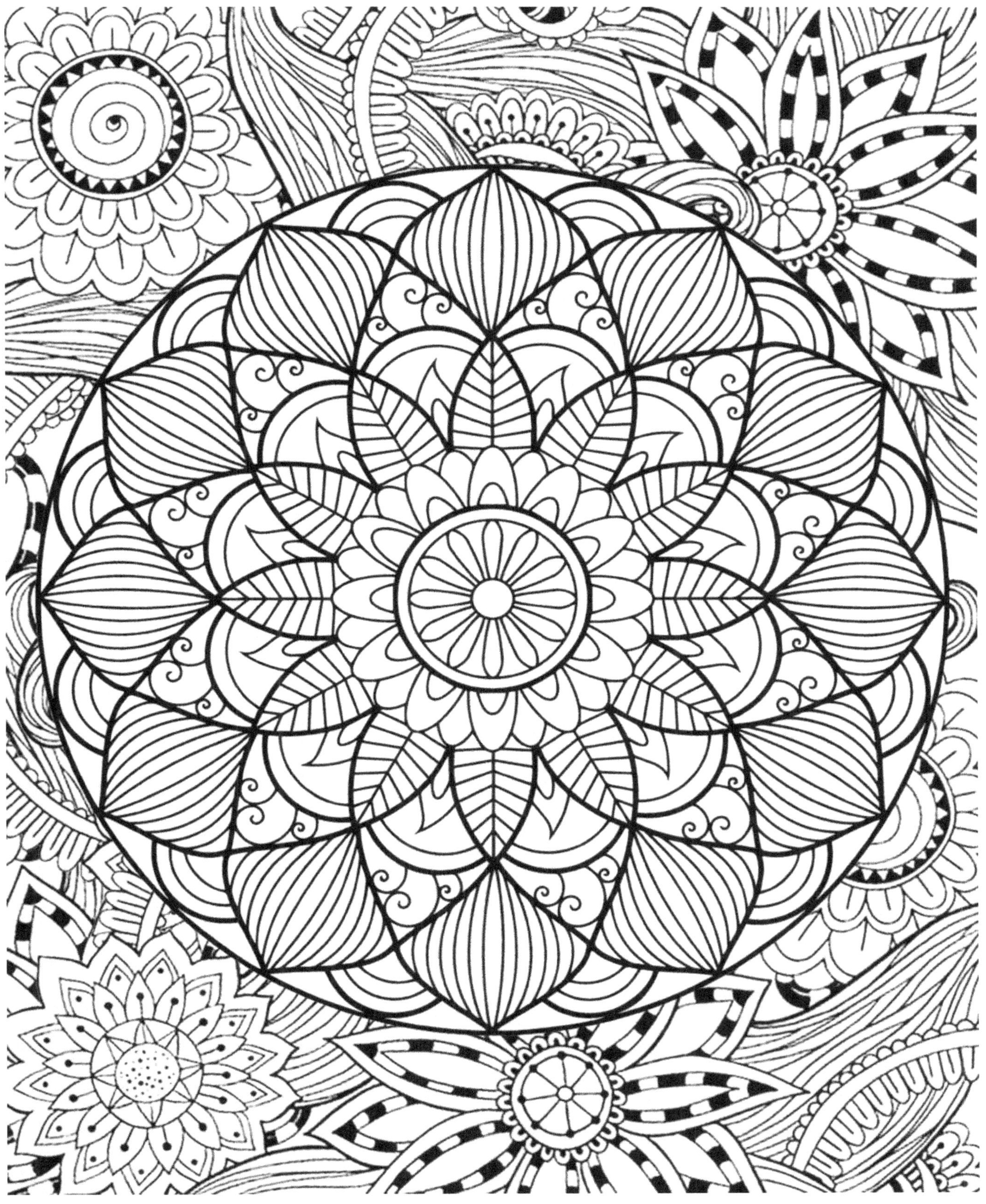

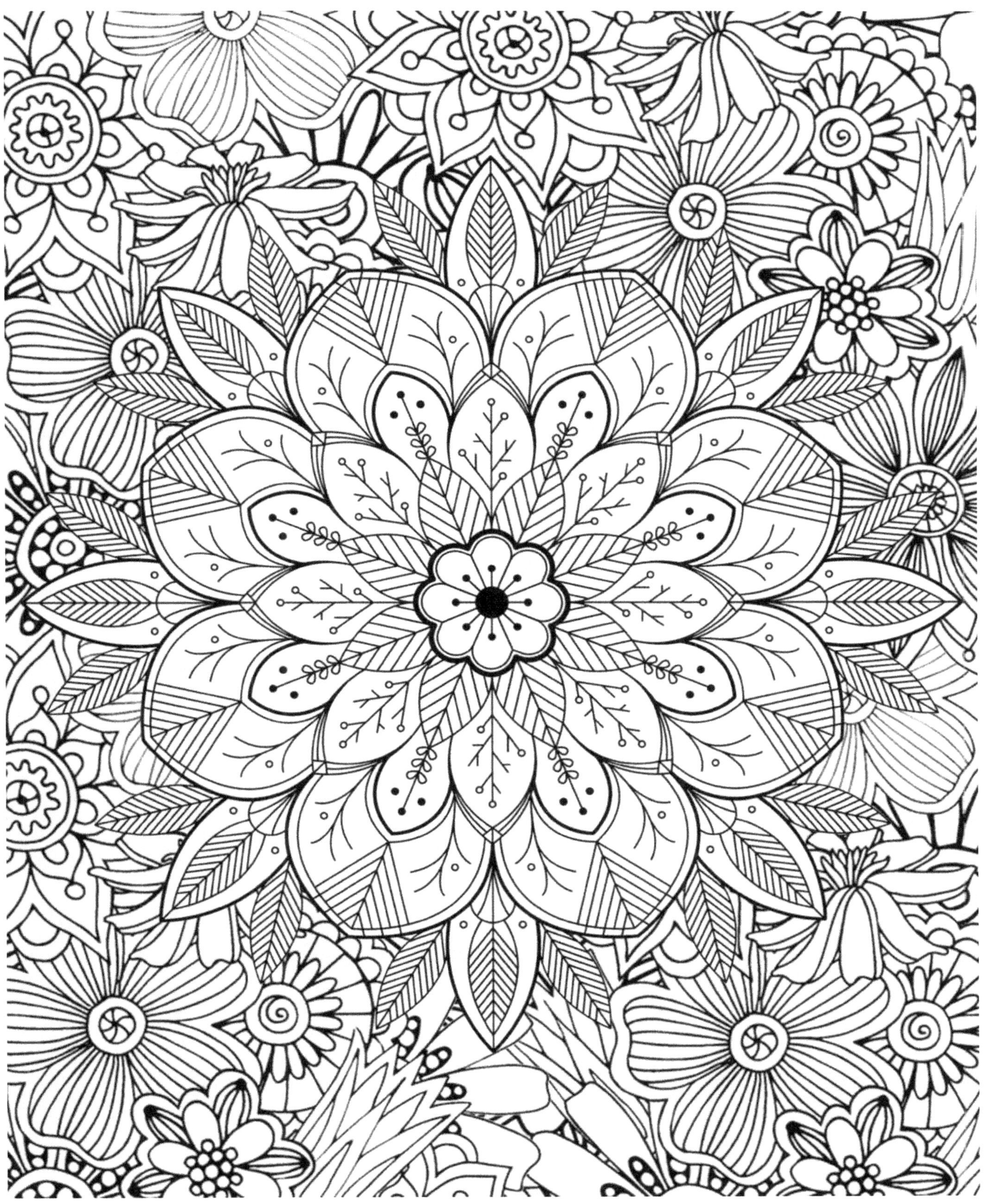

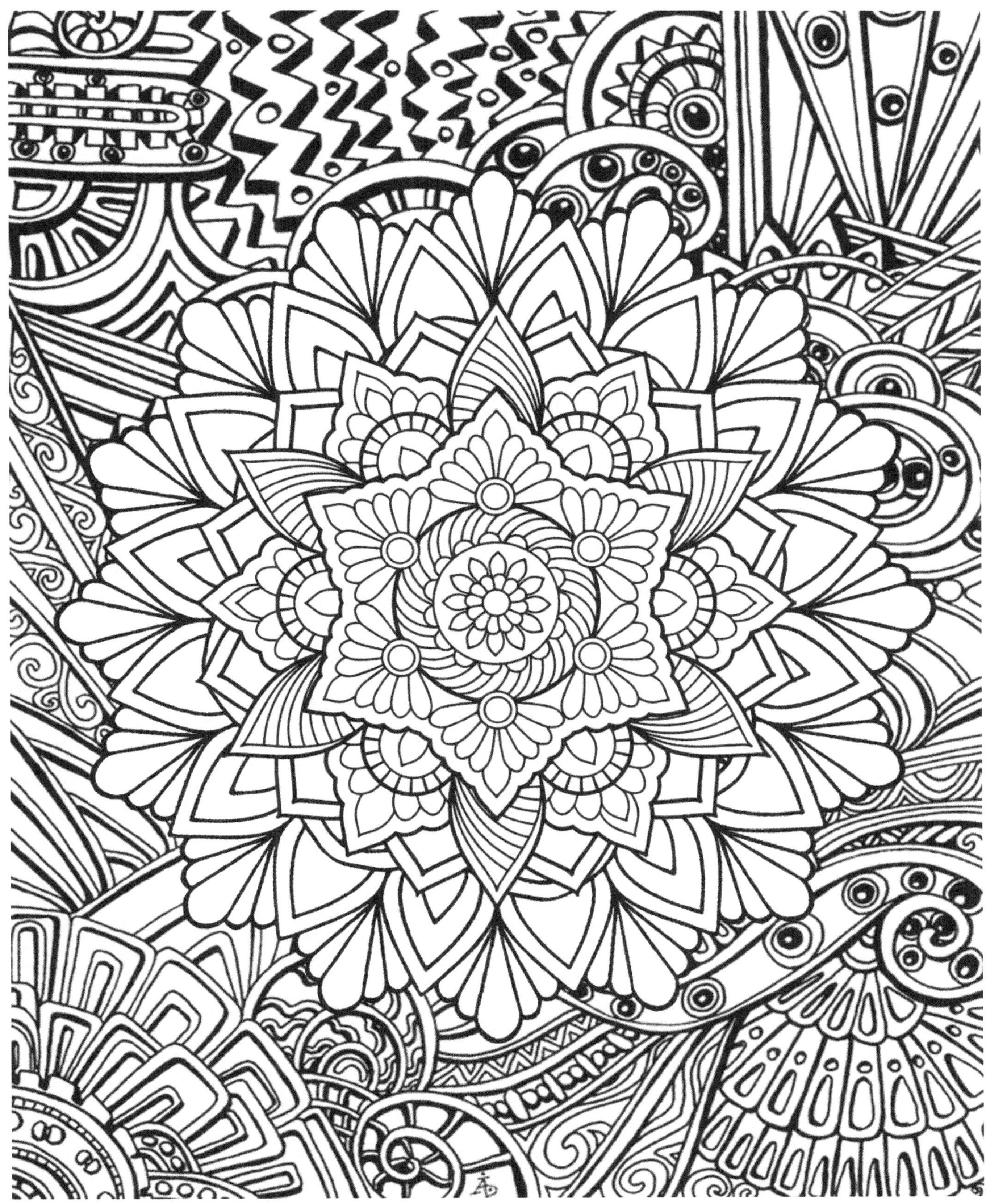

 

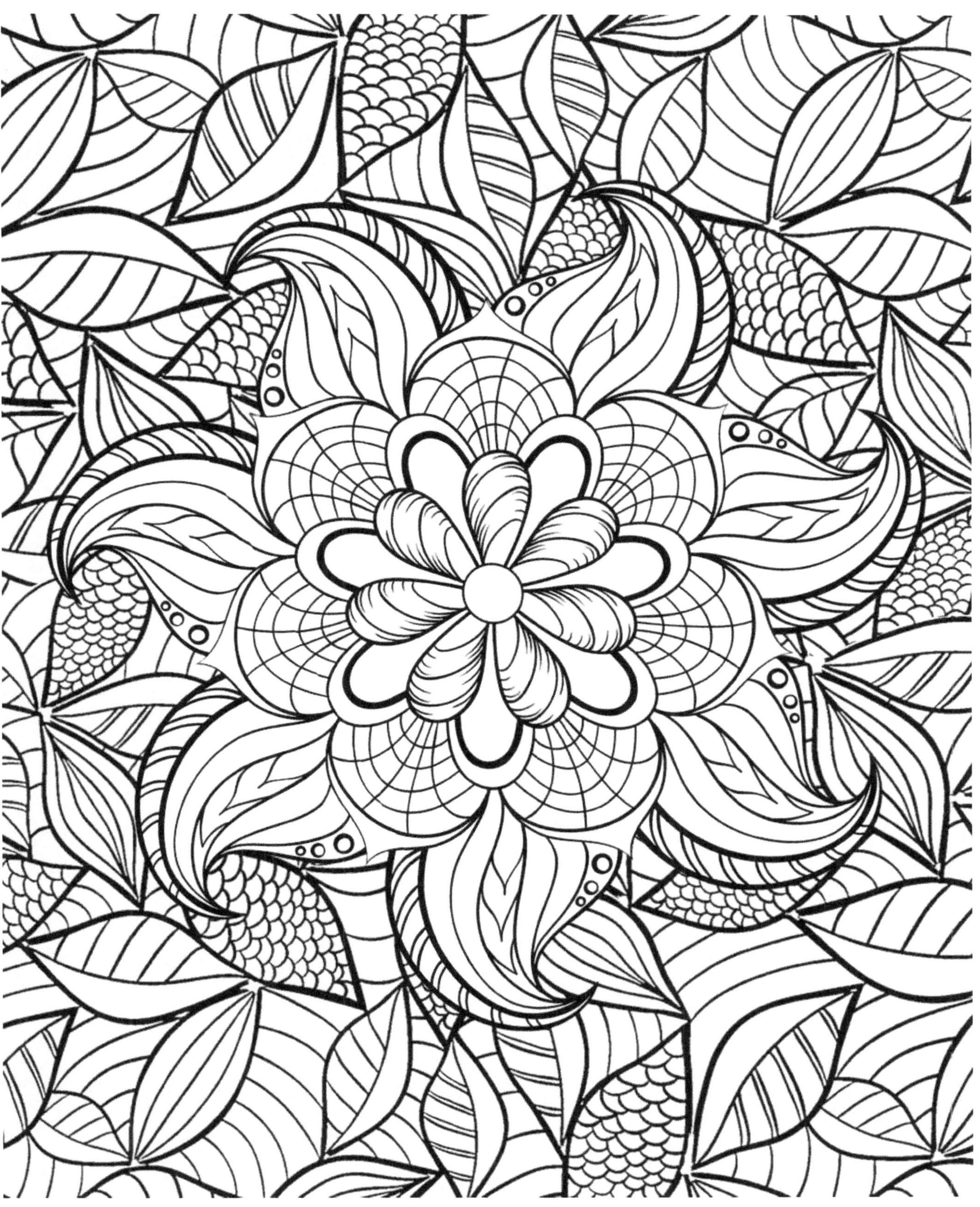

 

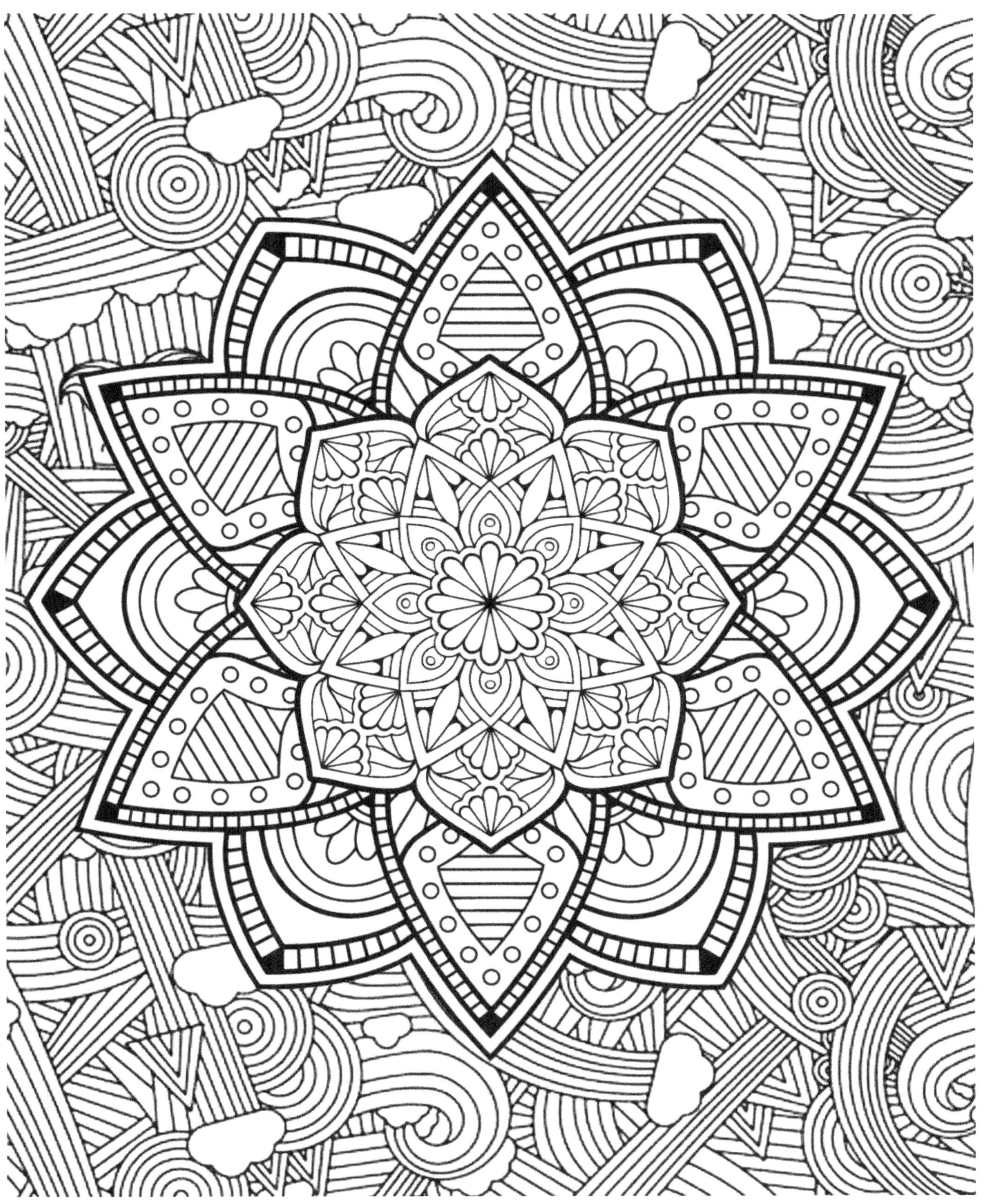

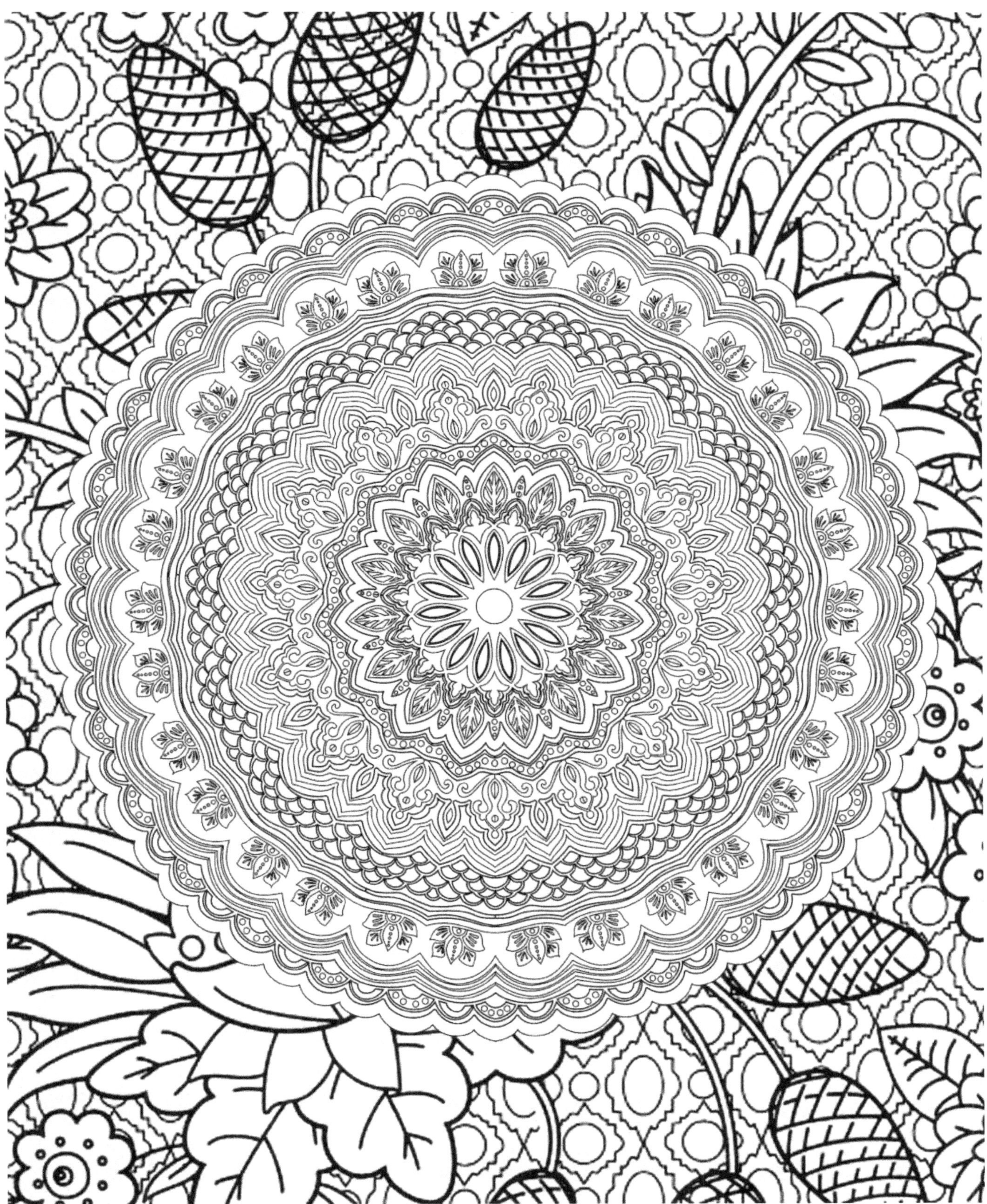

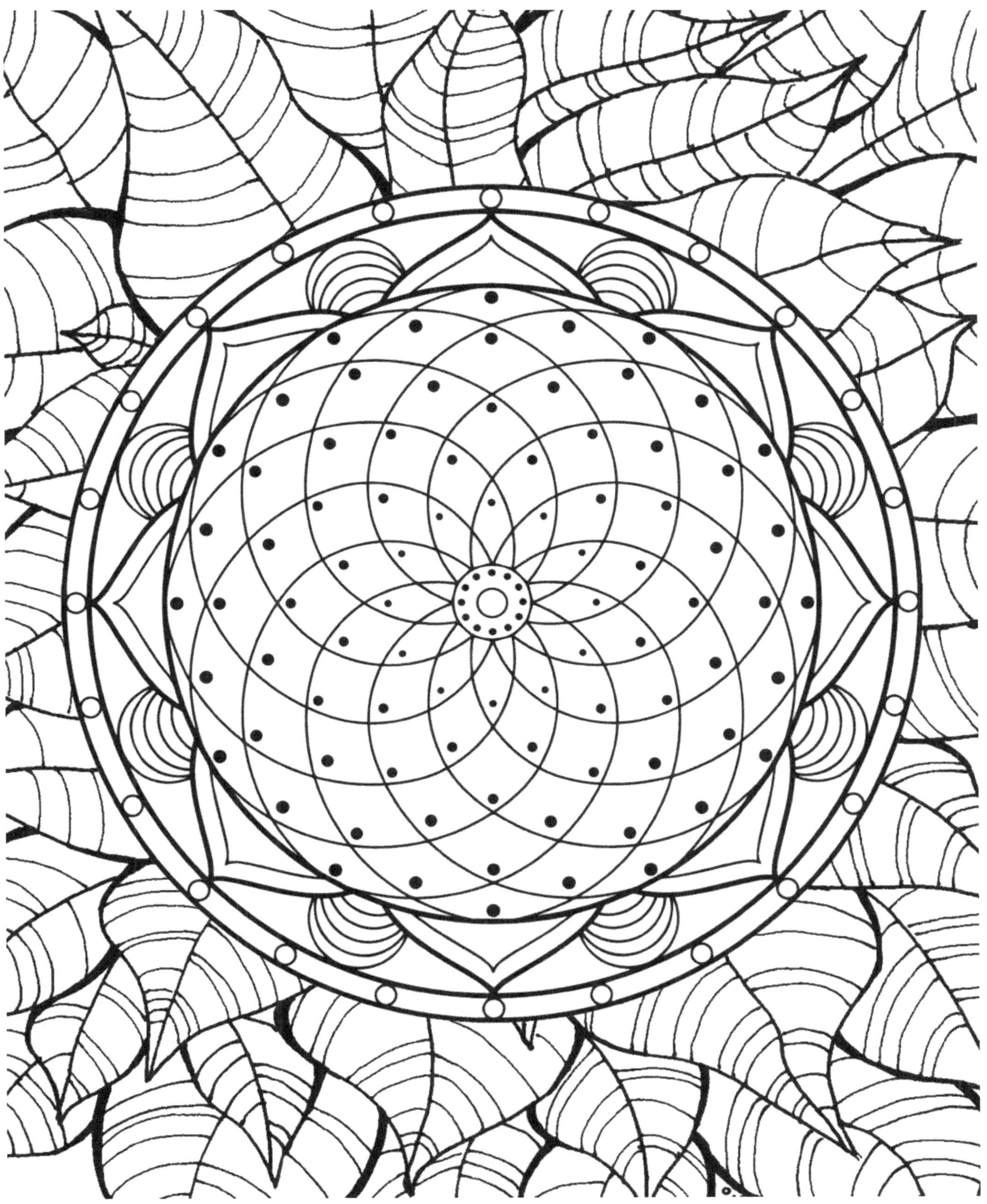

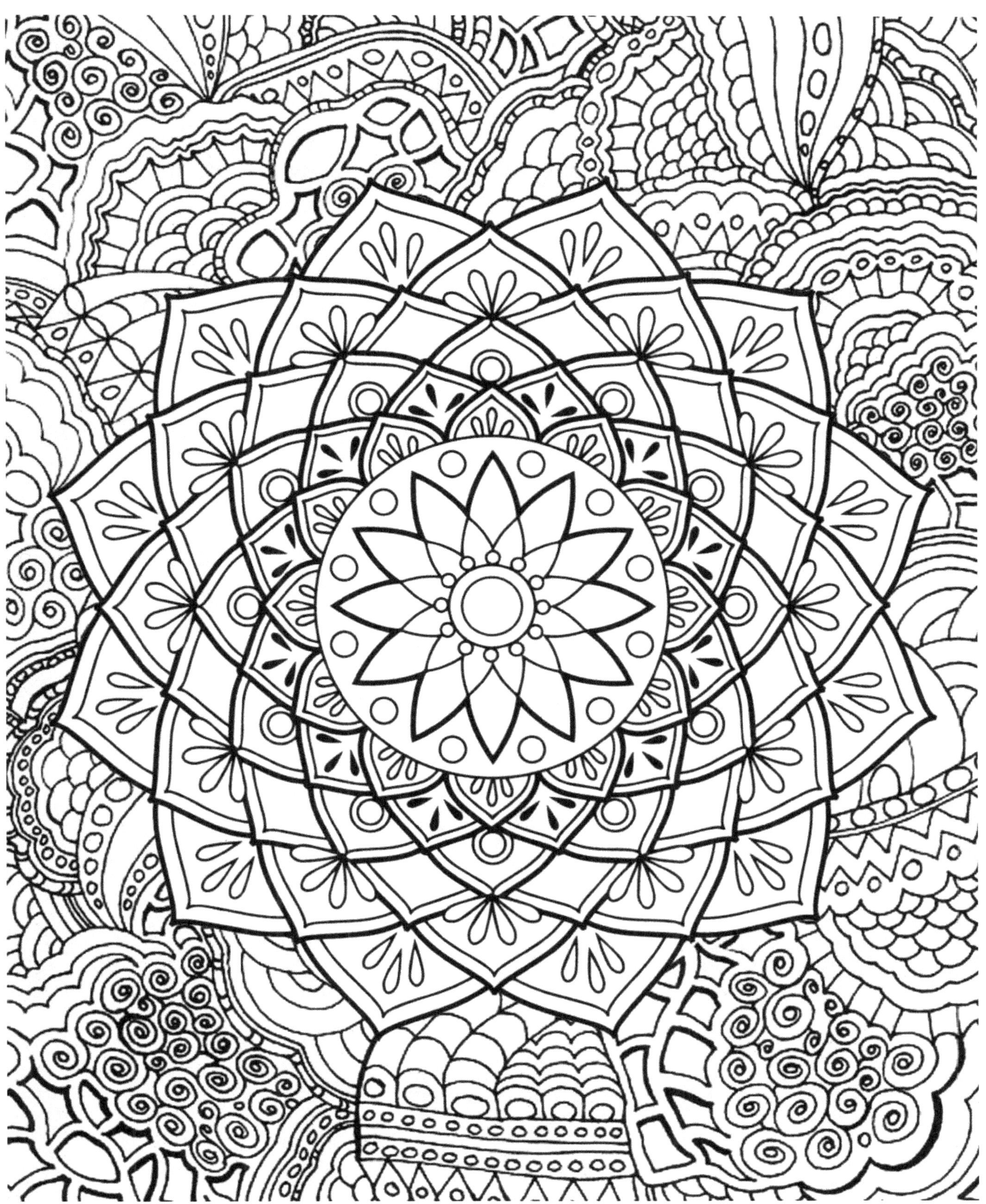

 

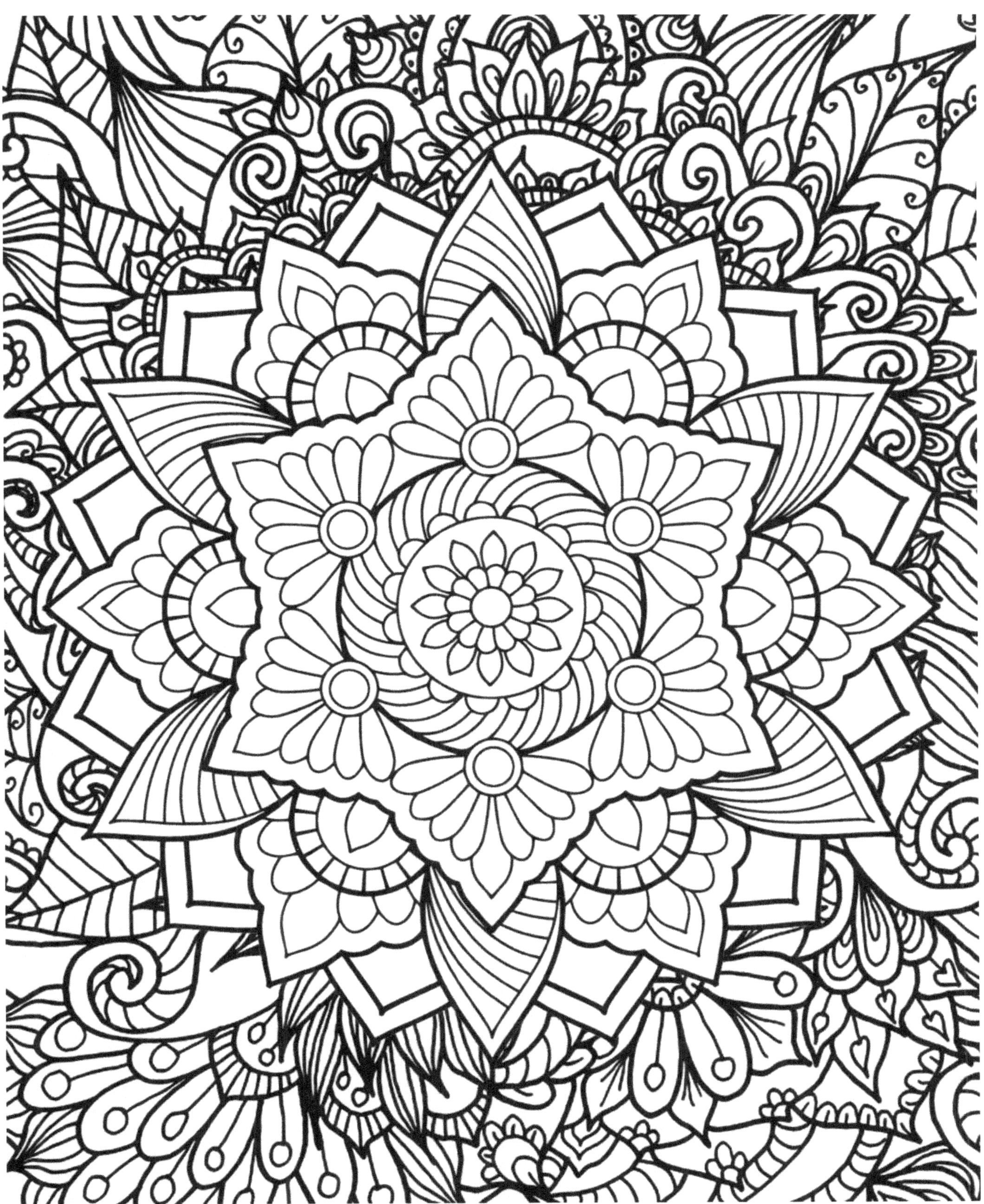

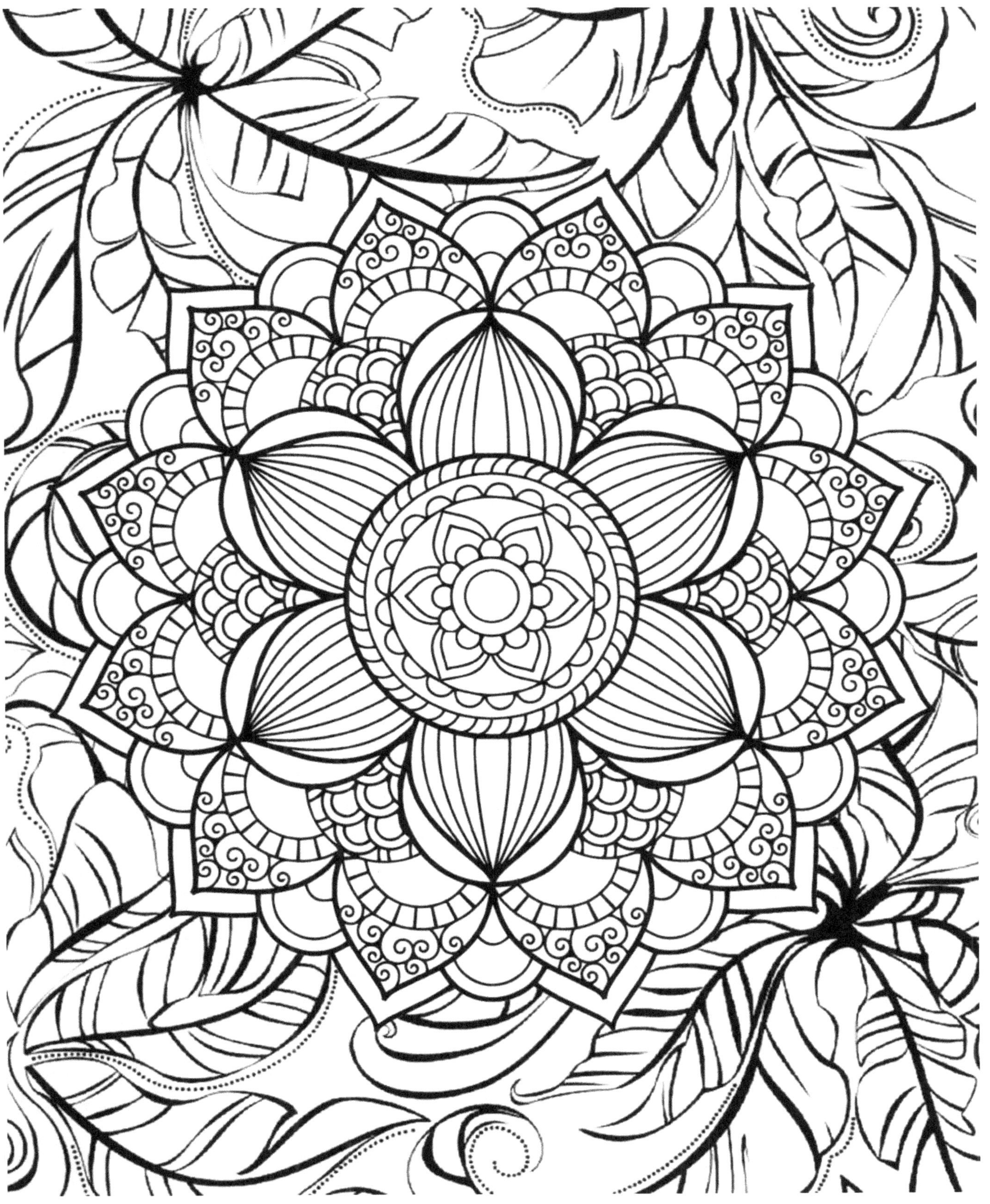

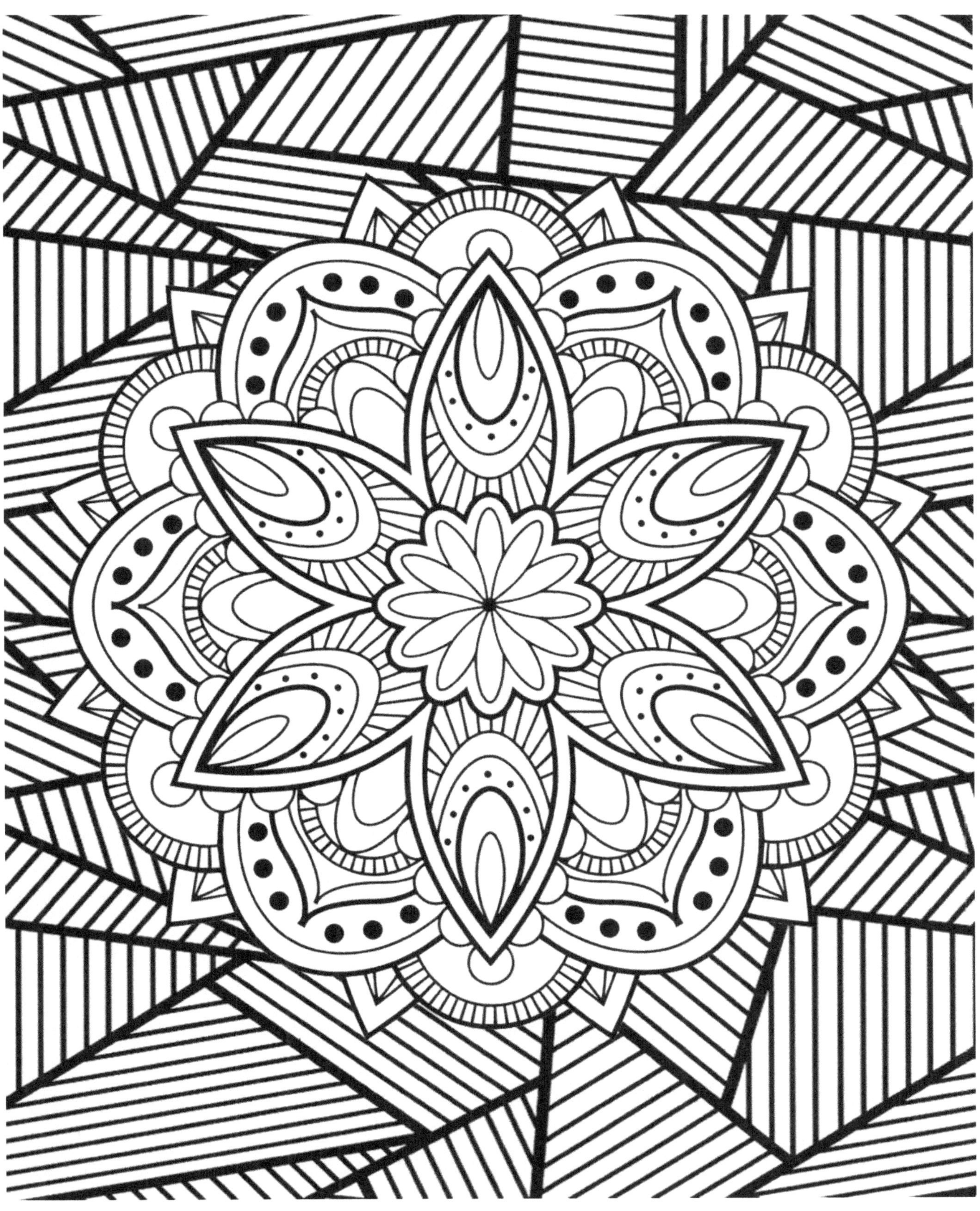

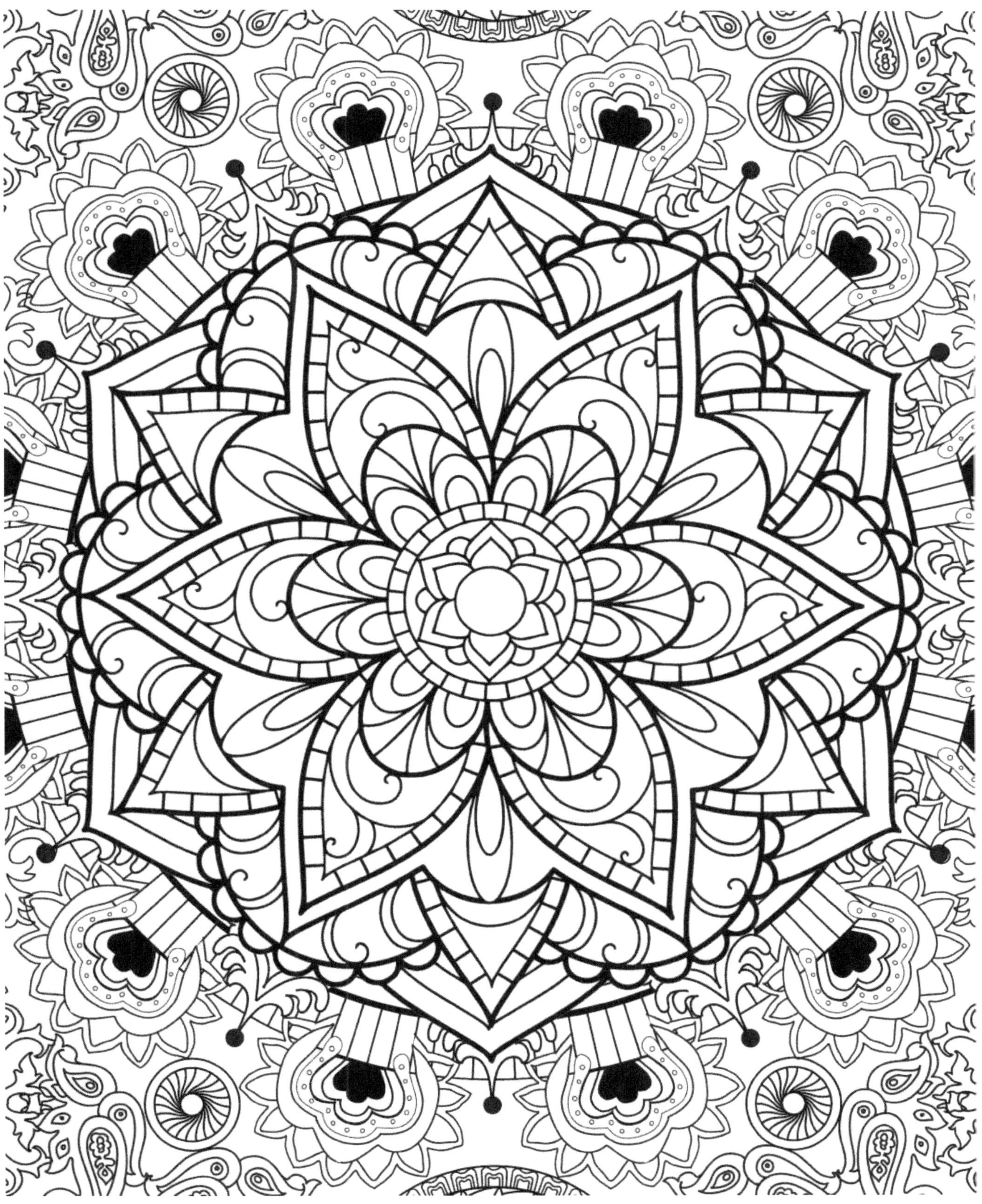

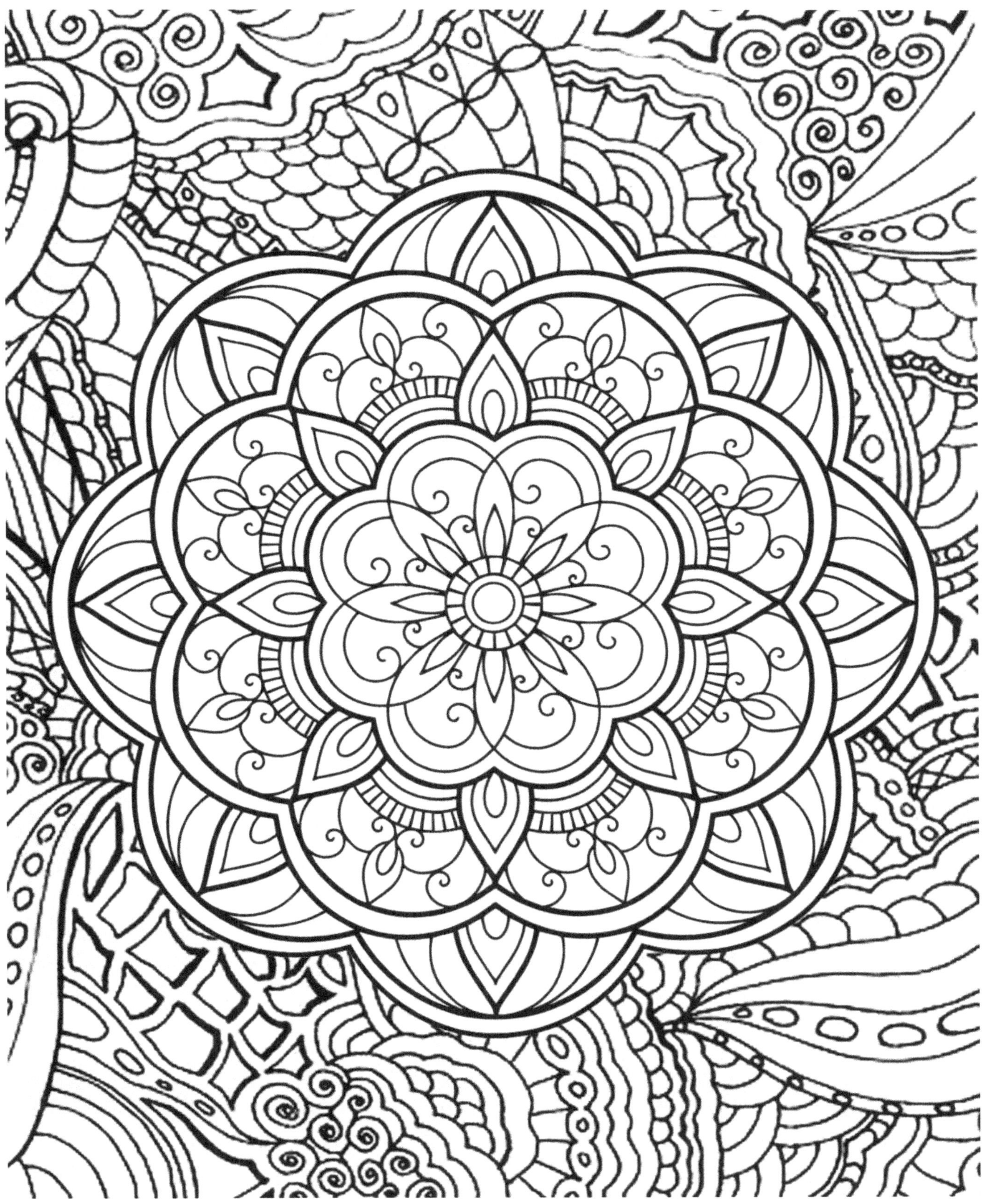

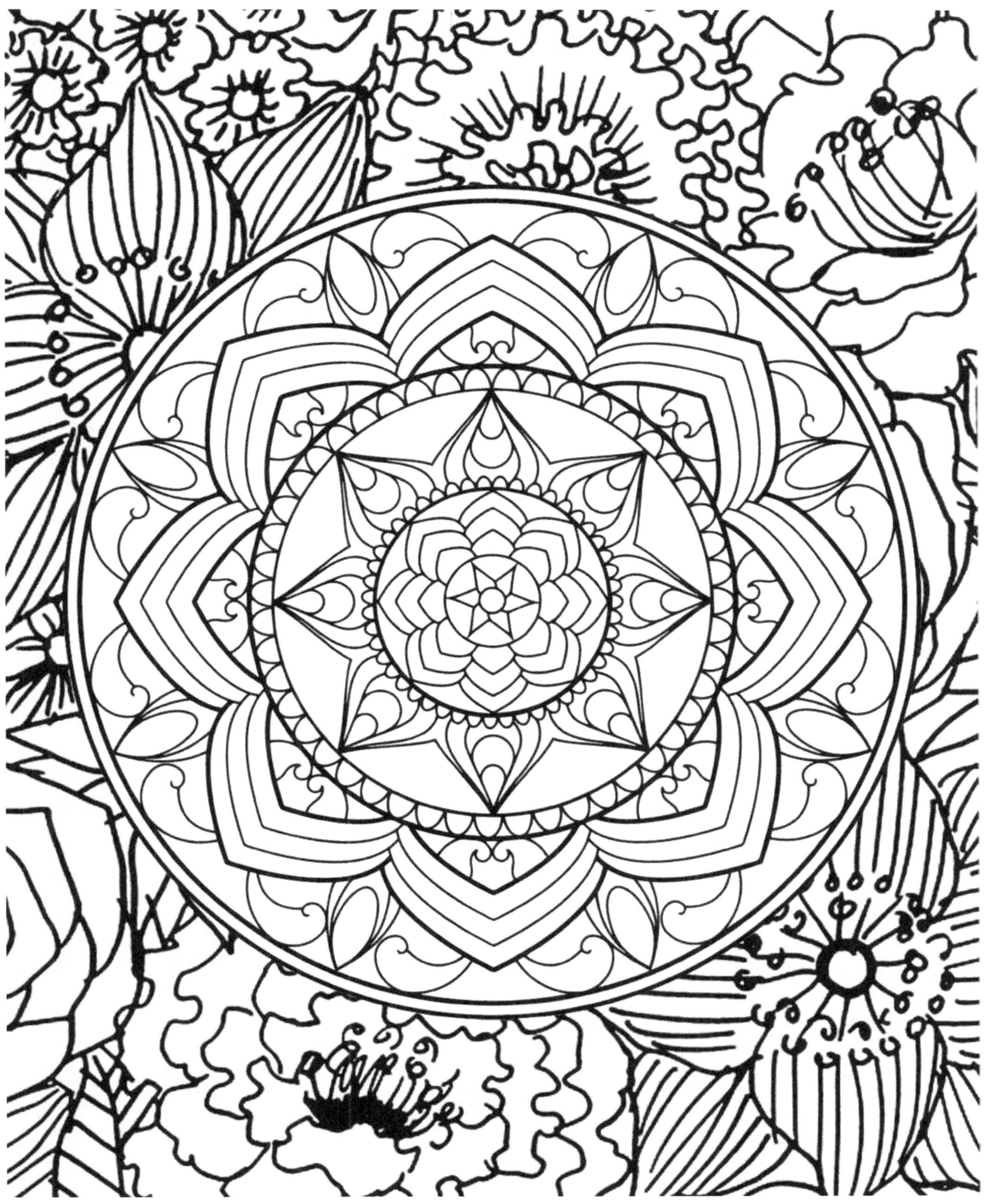

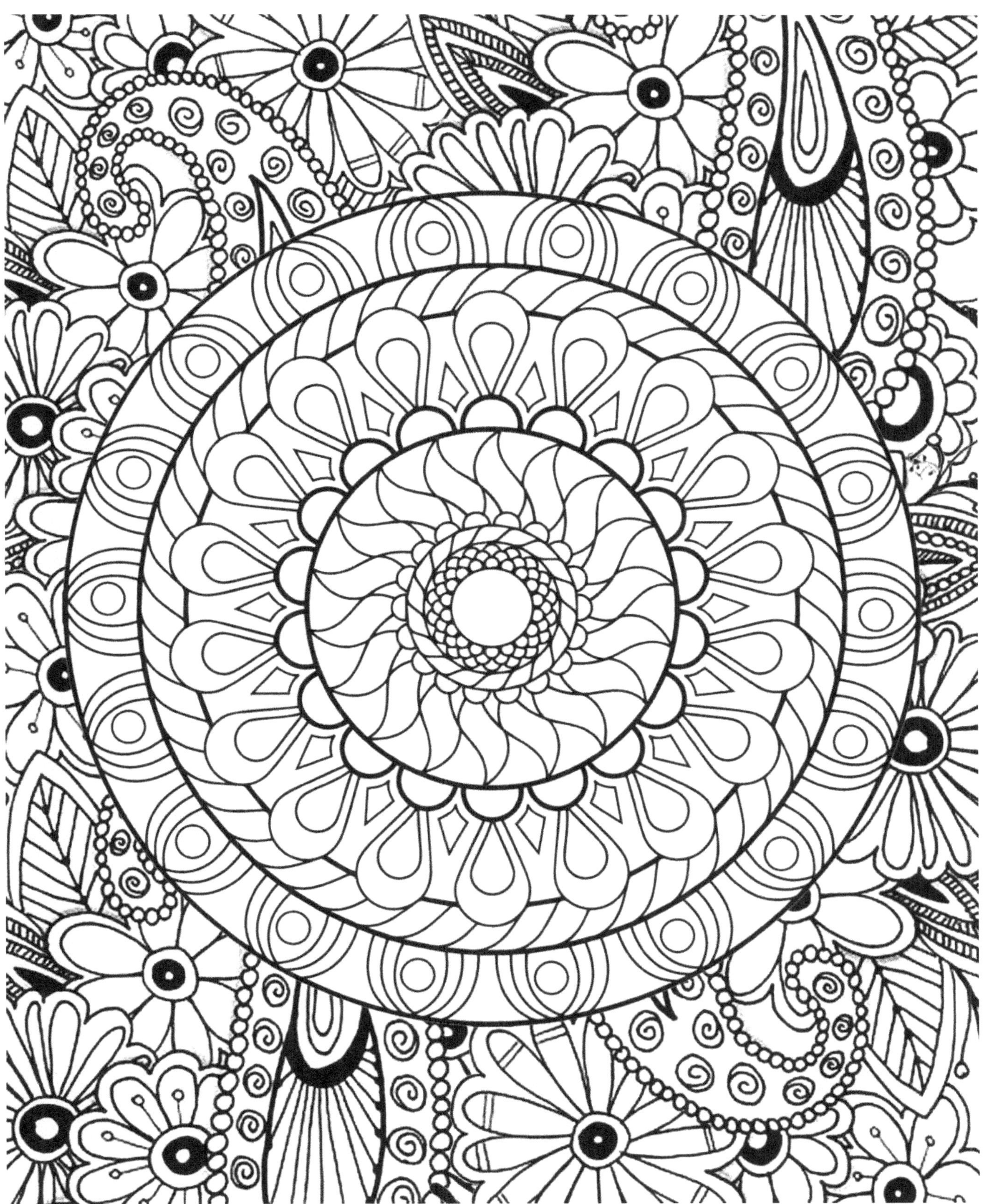

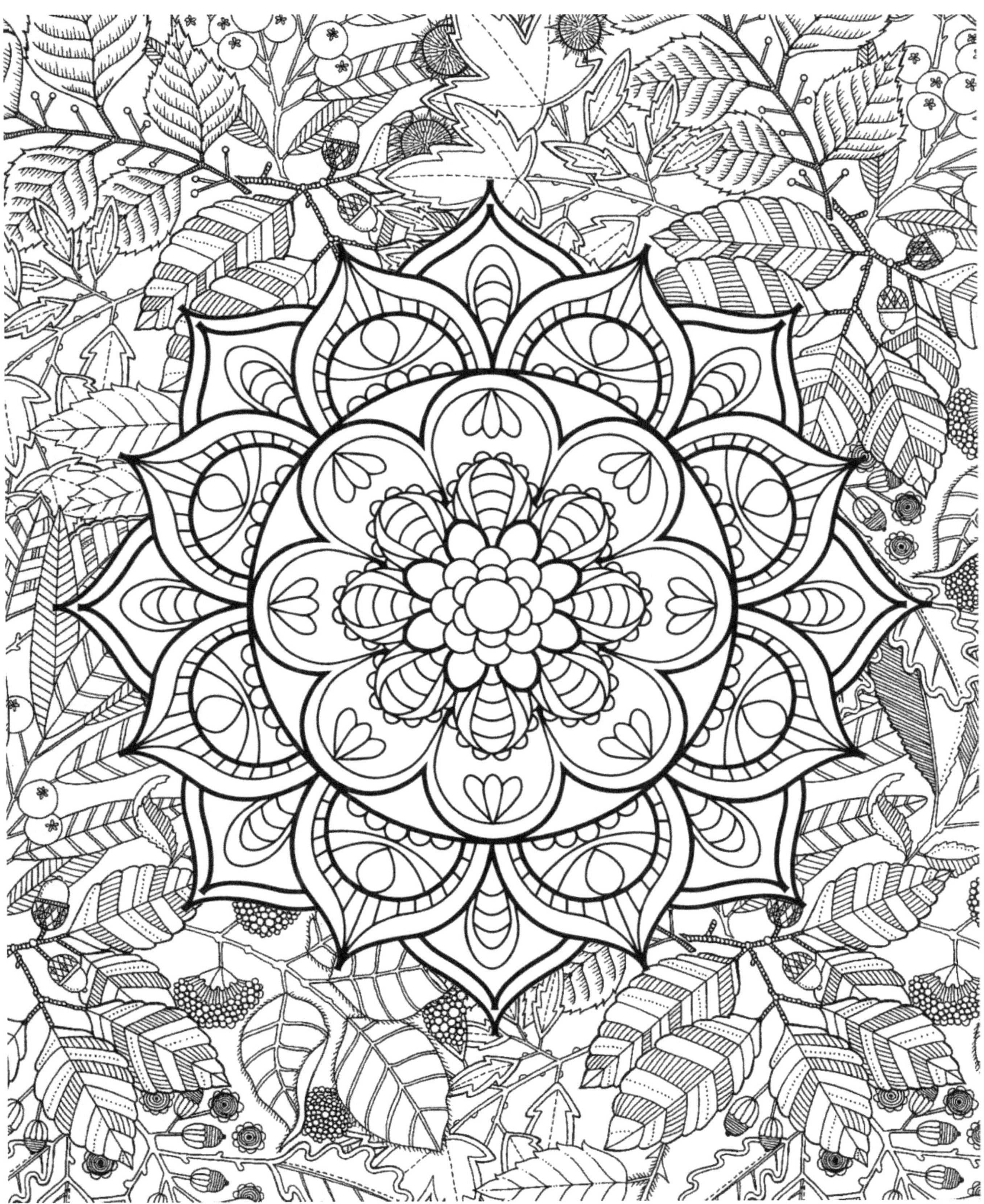

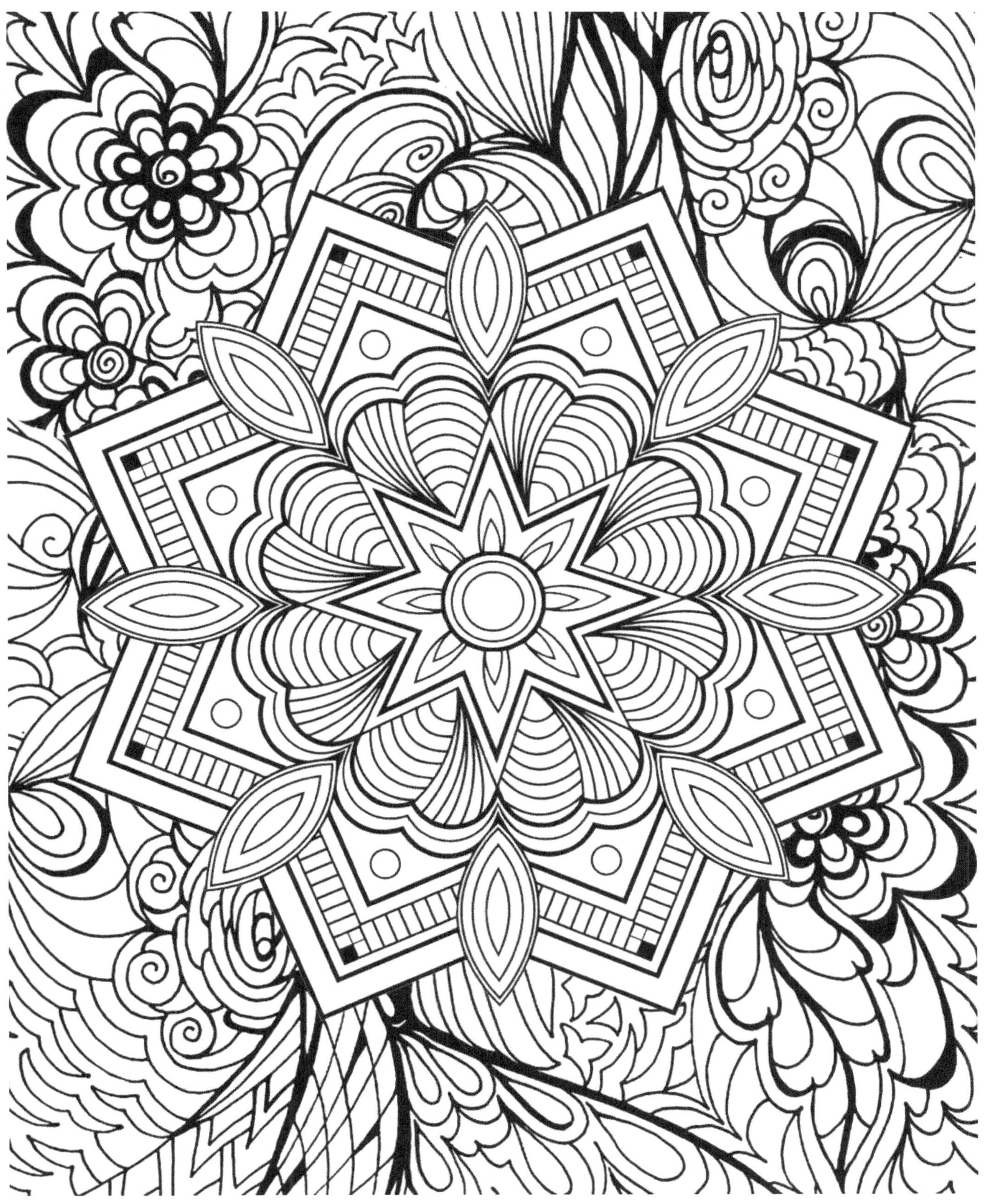

 

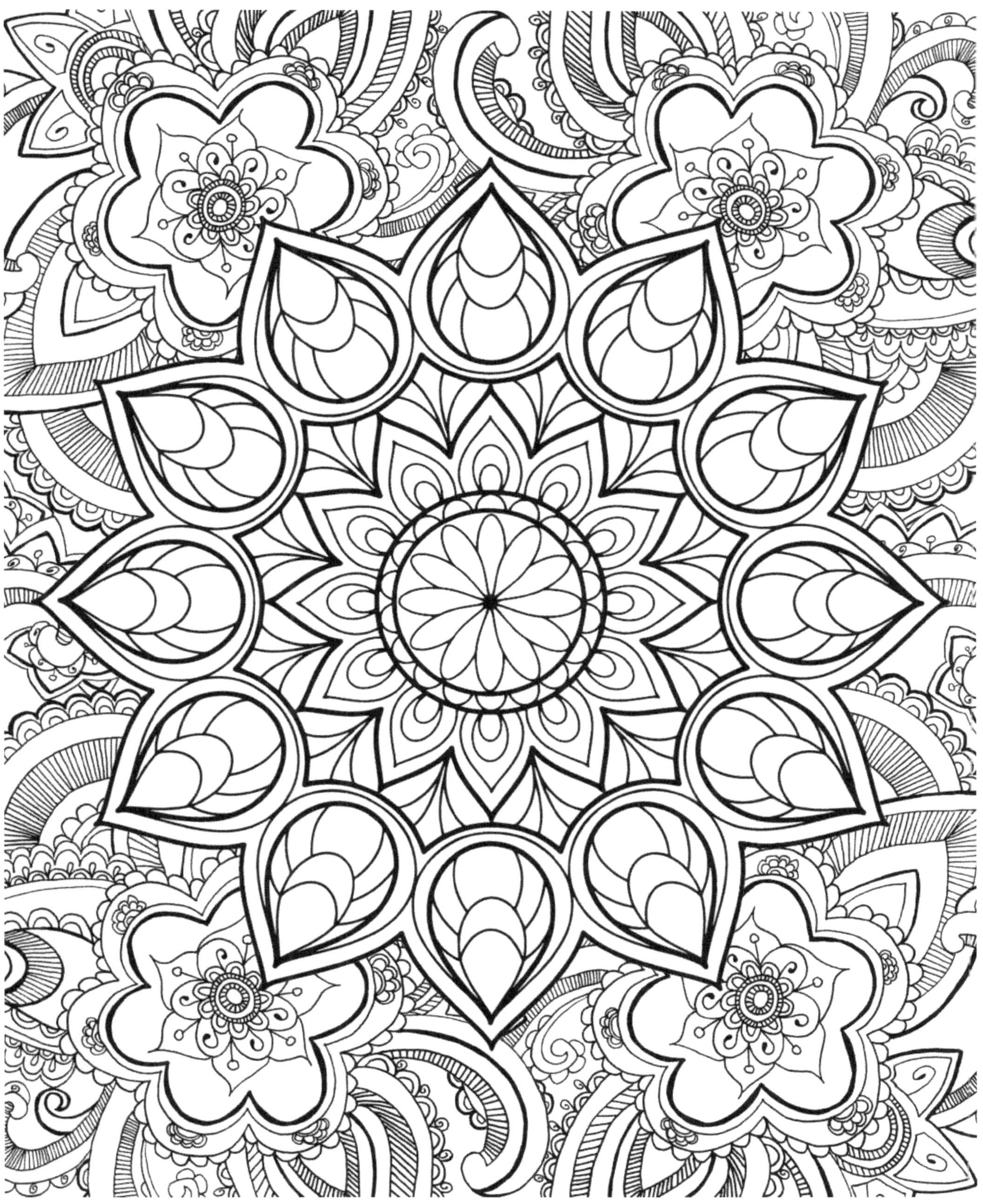

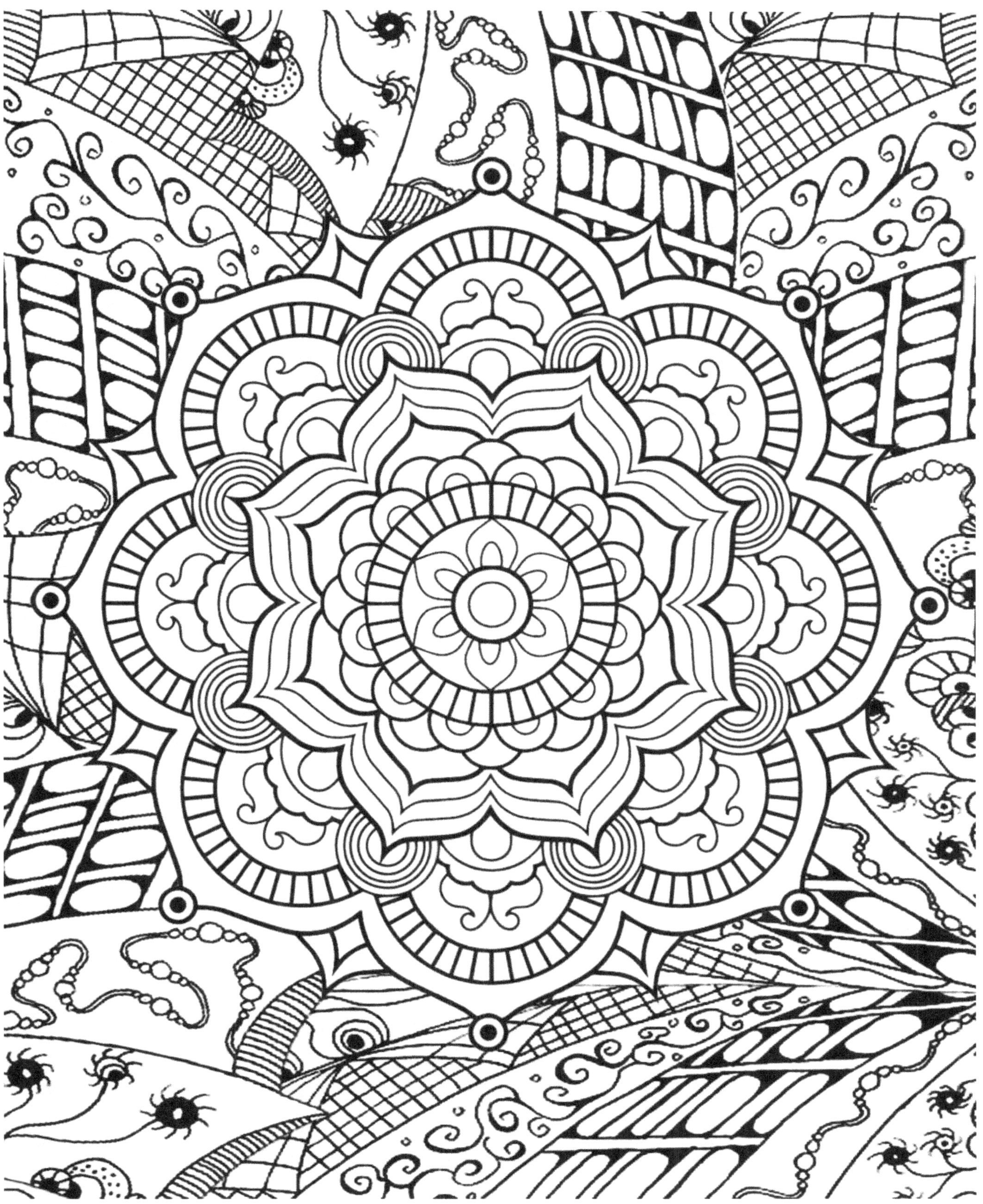

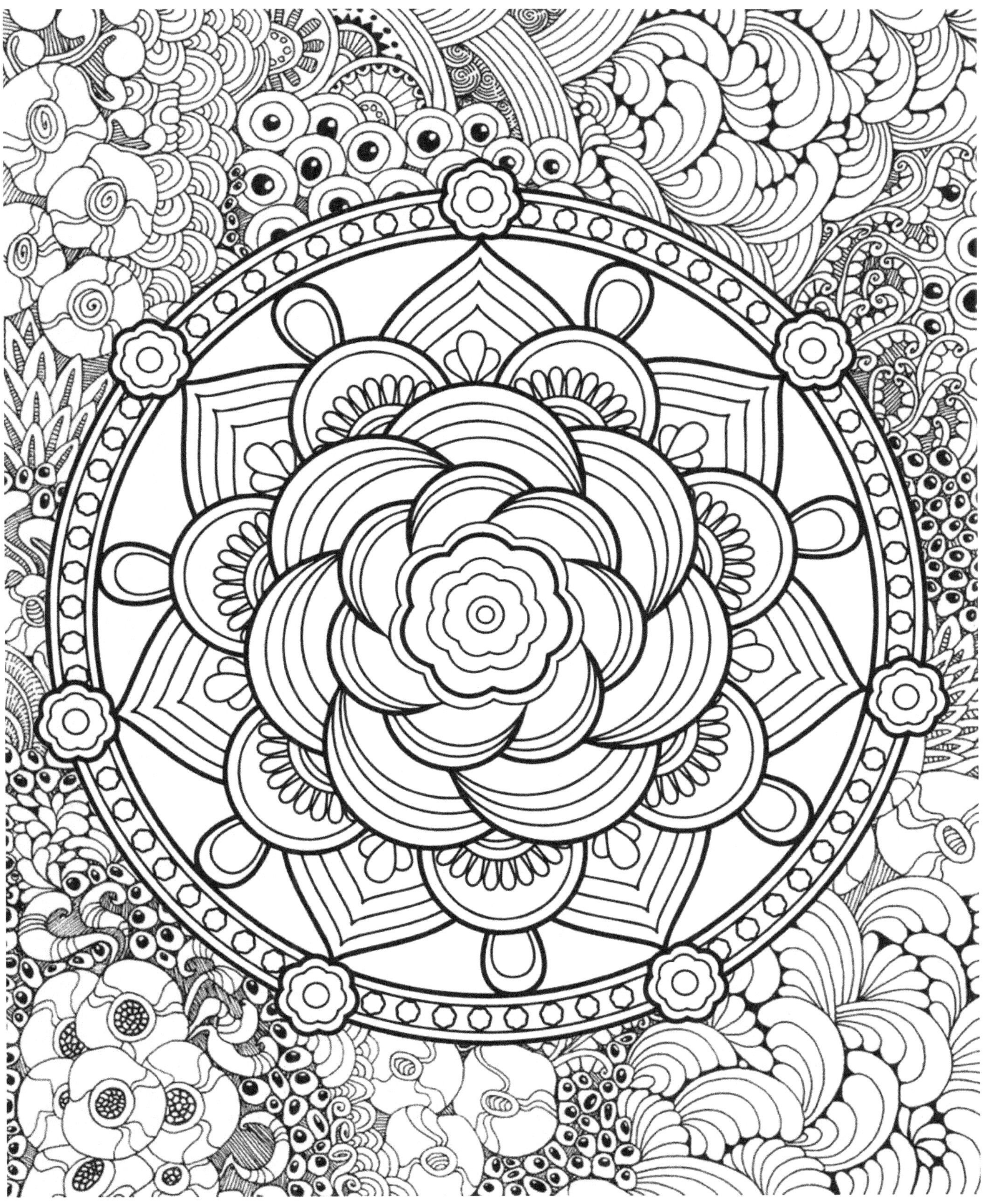

 

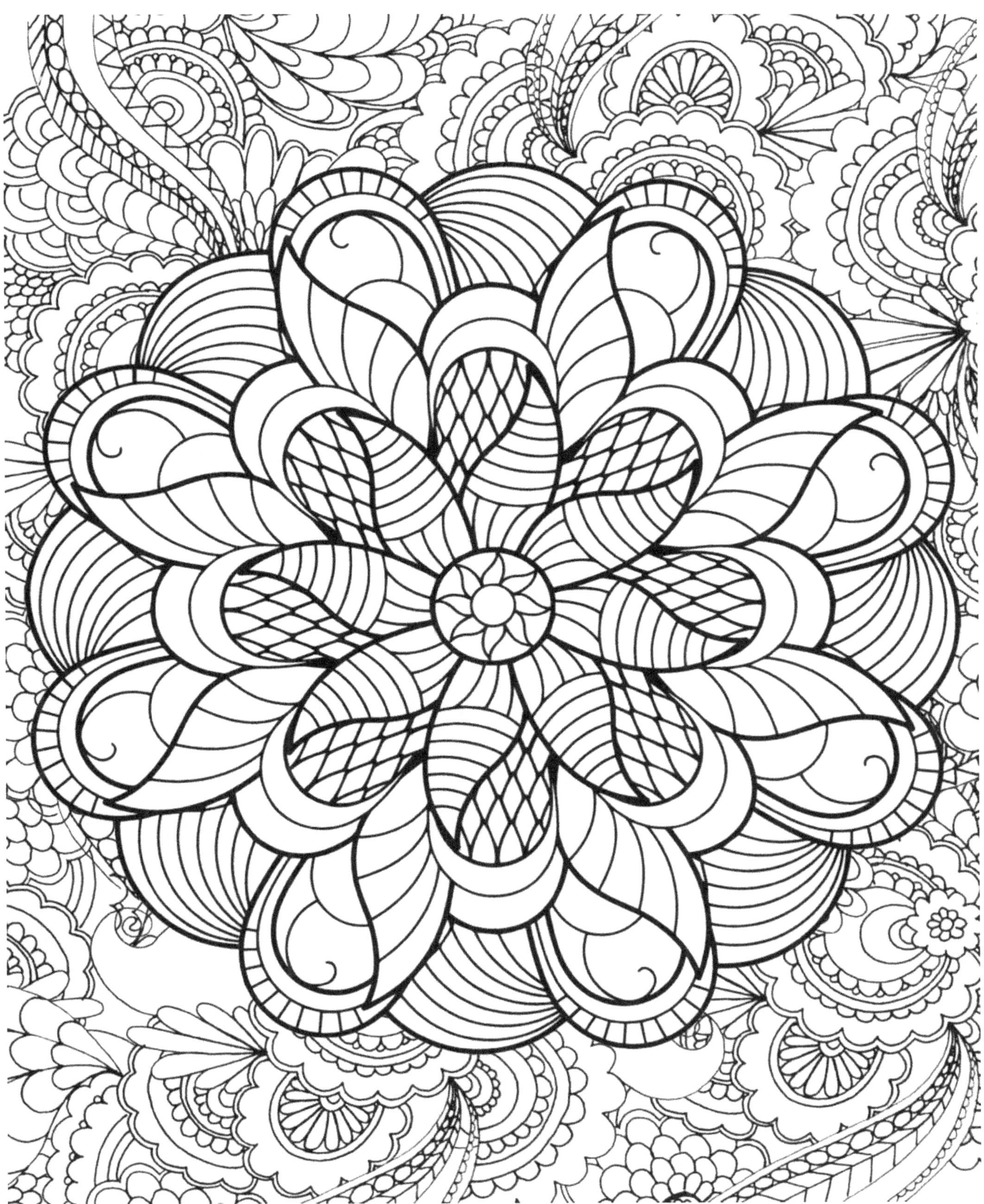

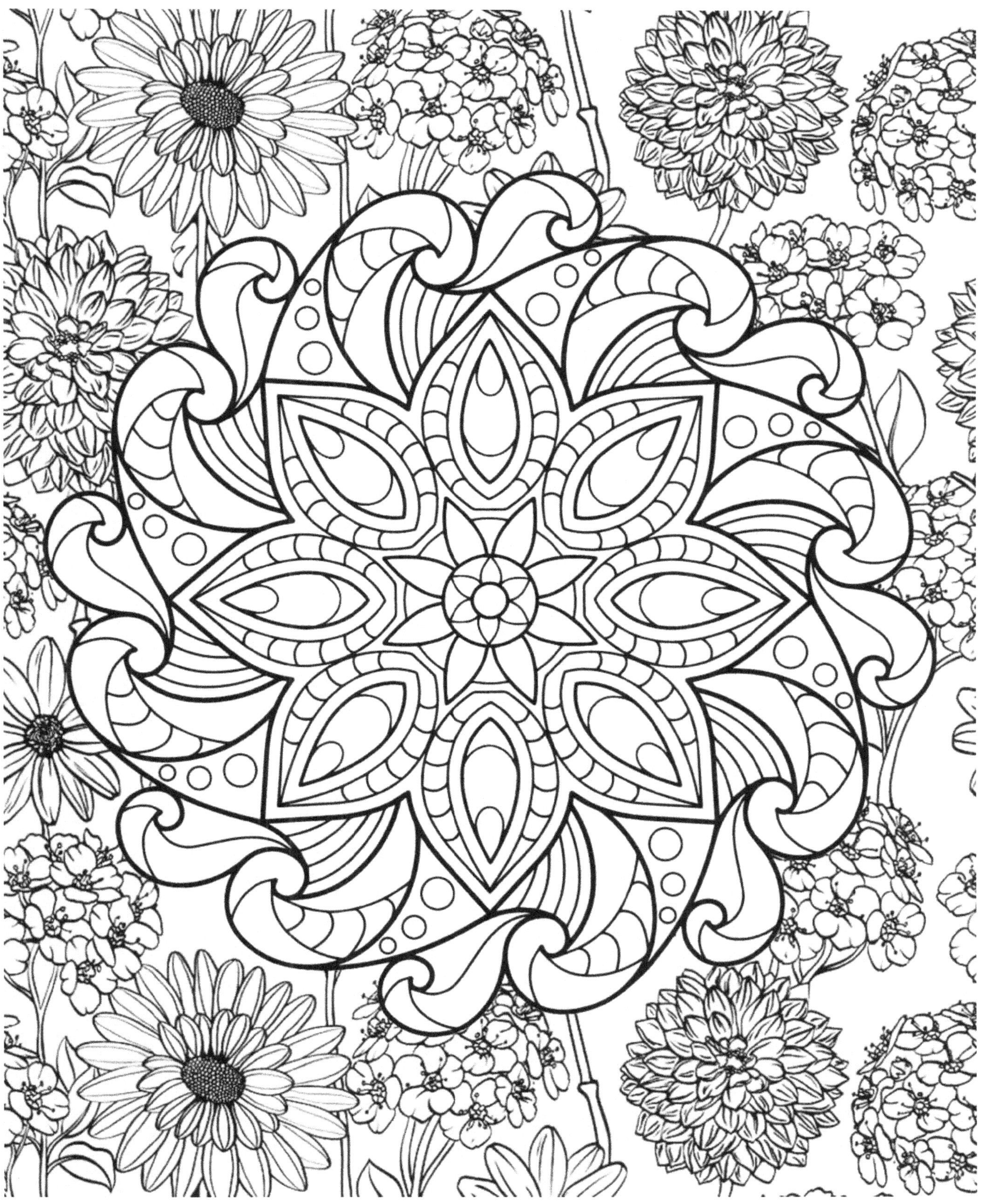

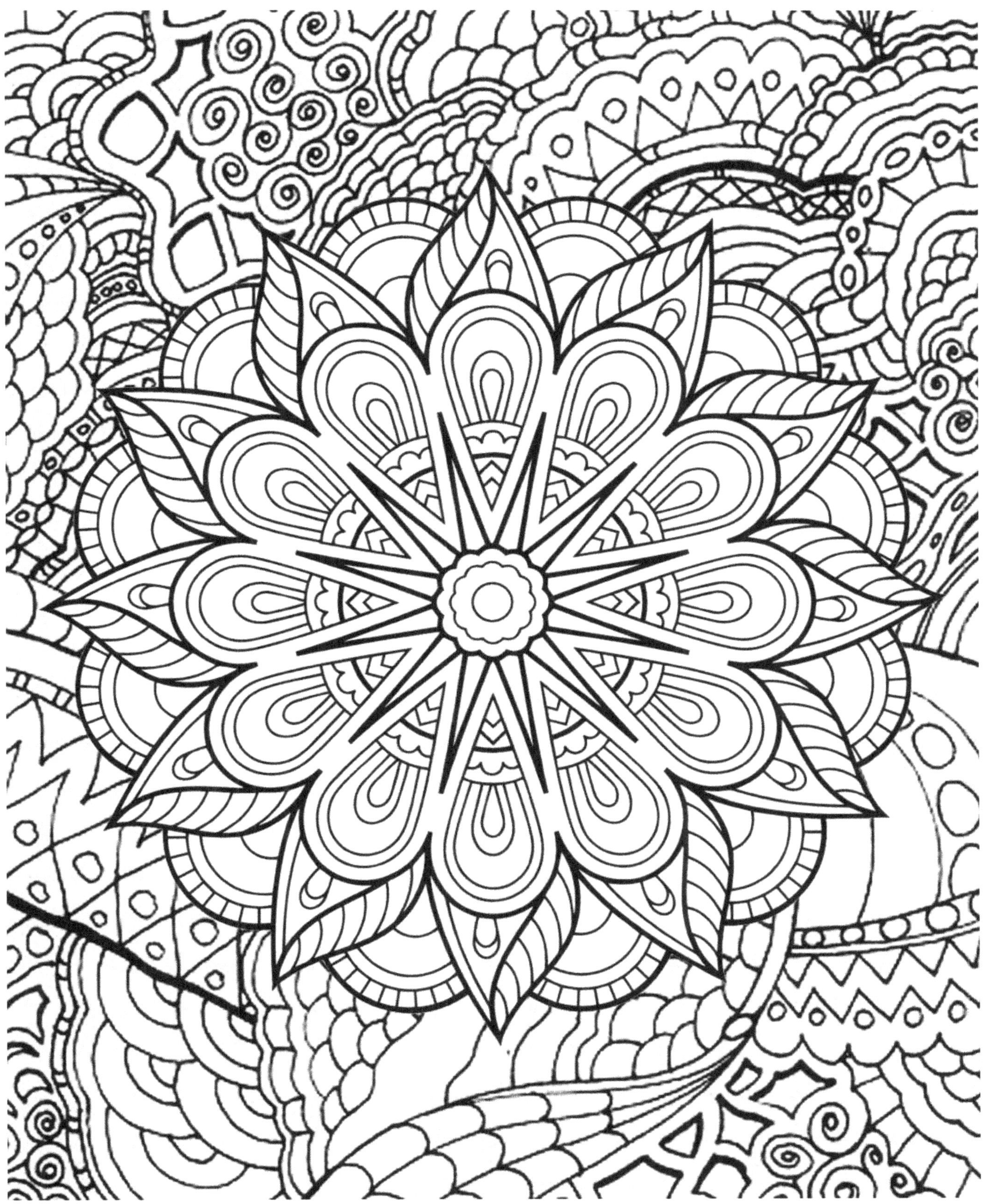

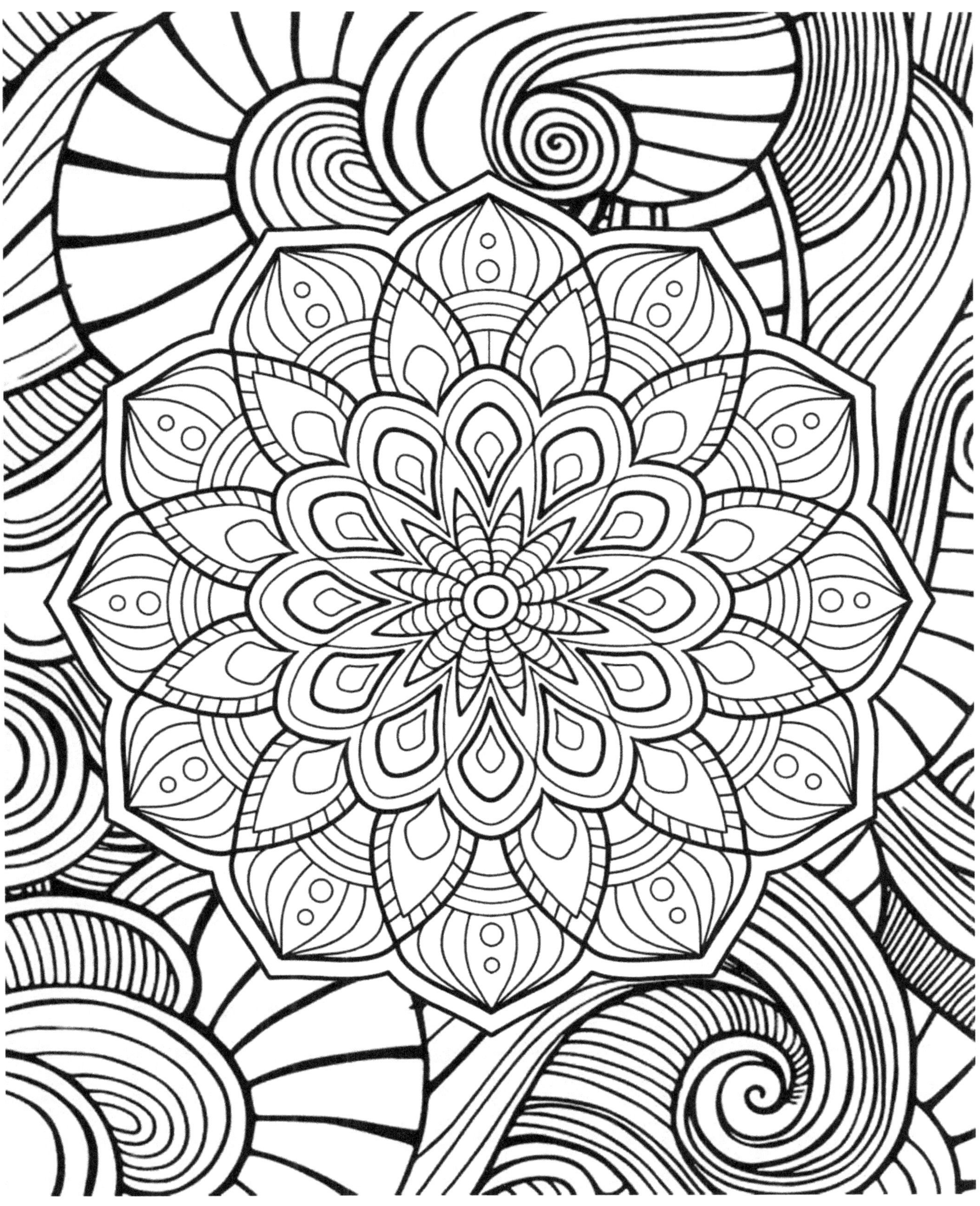

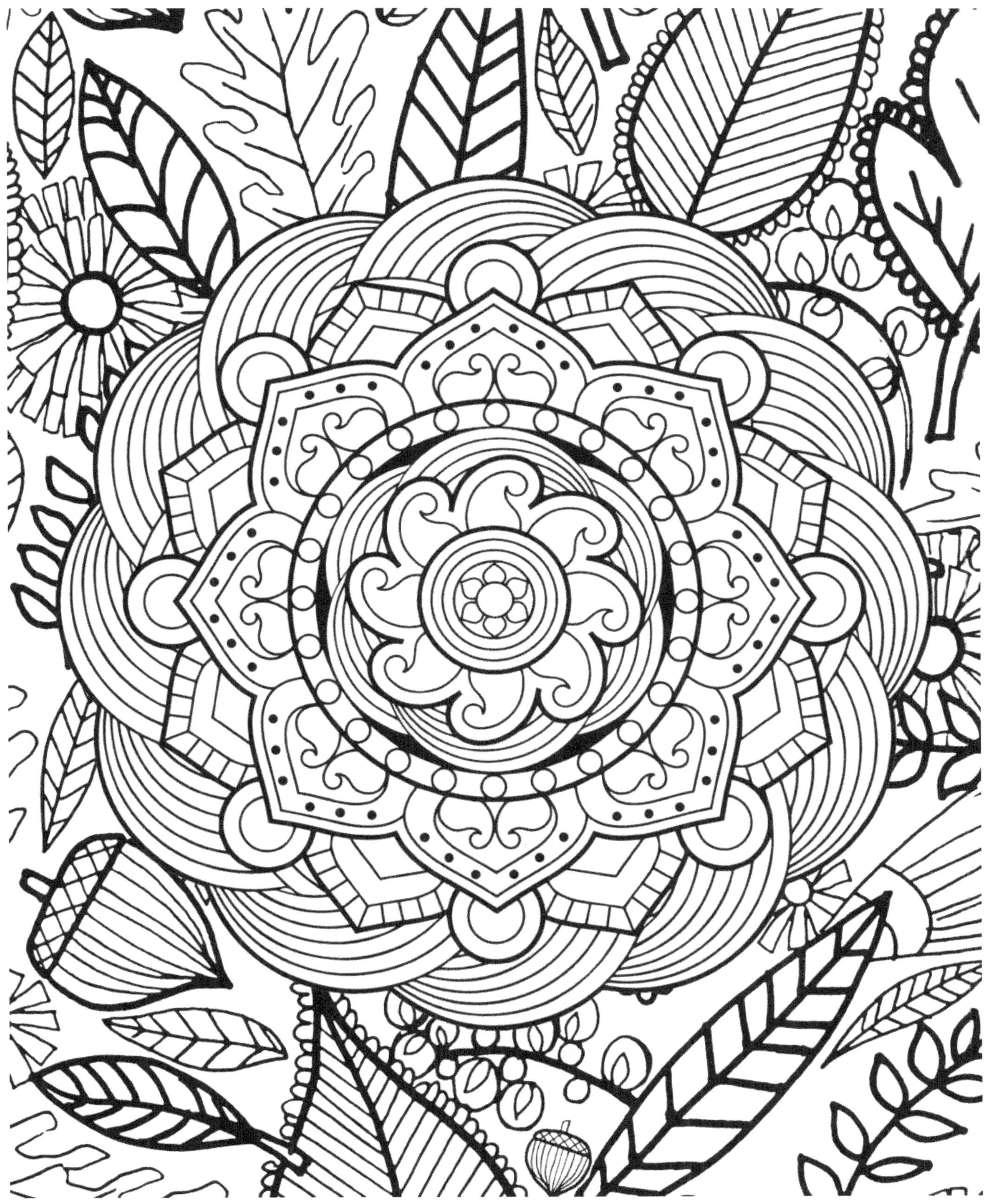

Mandala Coloring Book For Adult Art Therapy Anti Stress     Lenka Sarkhelova

 

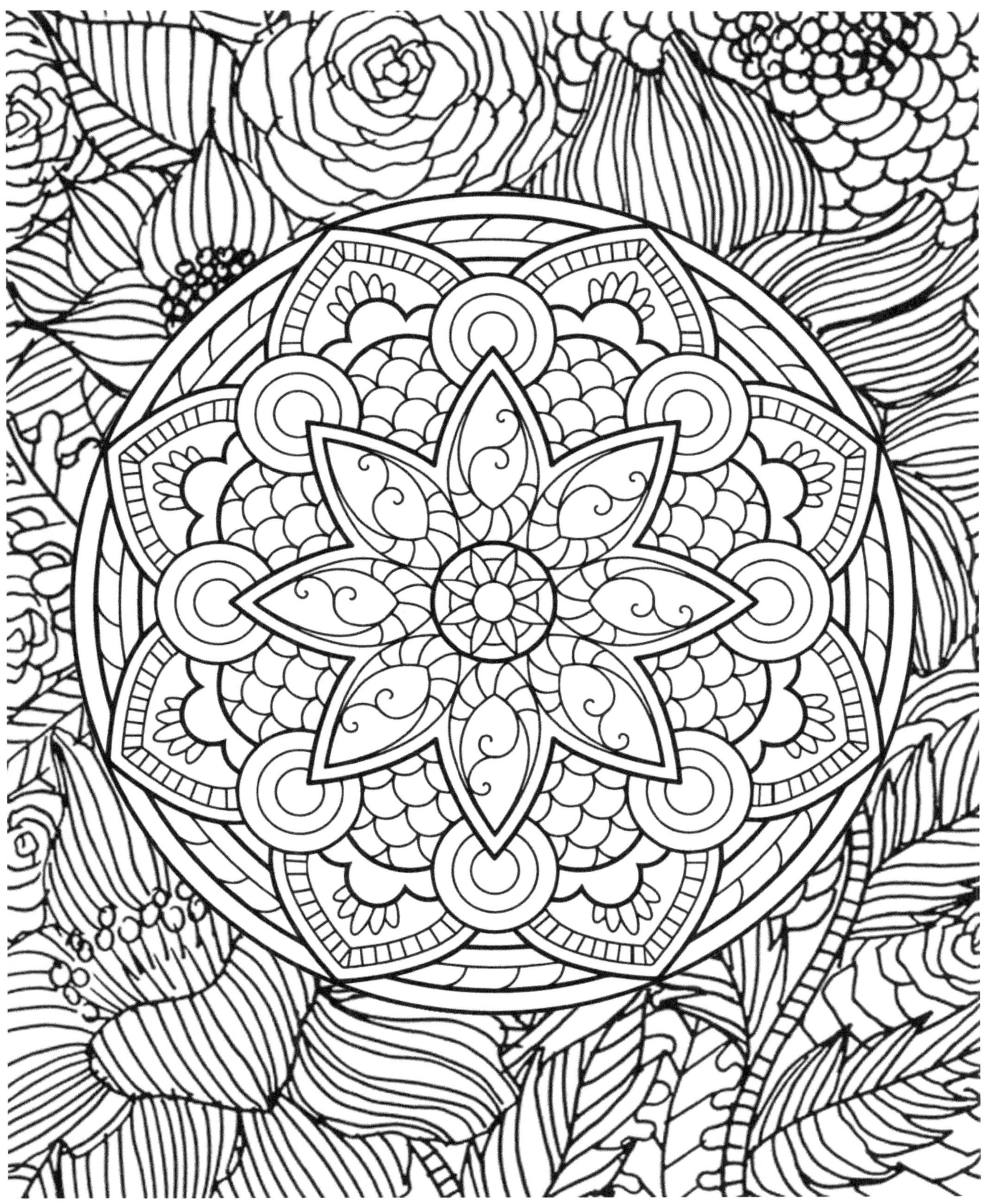

 

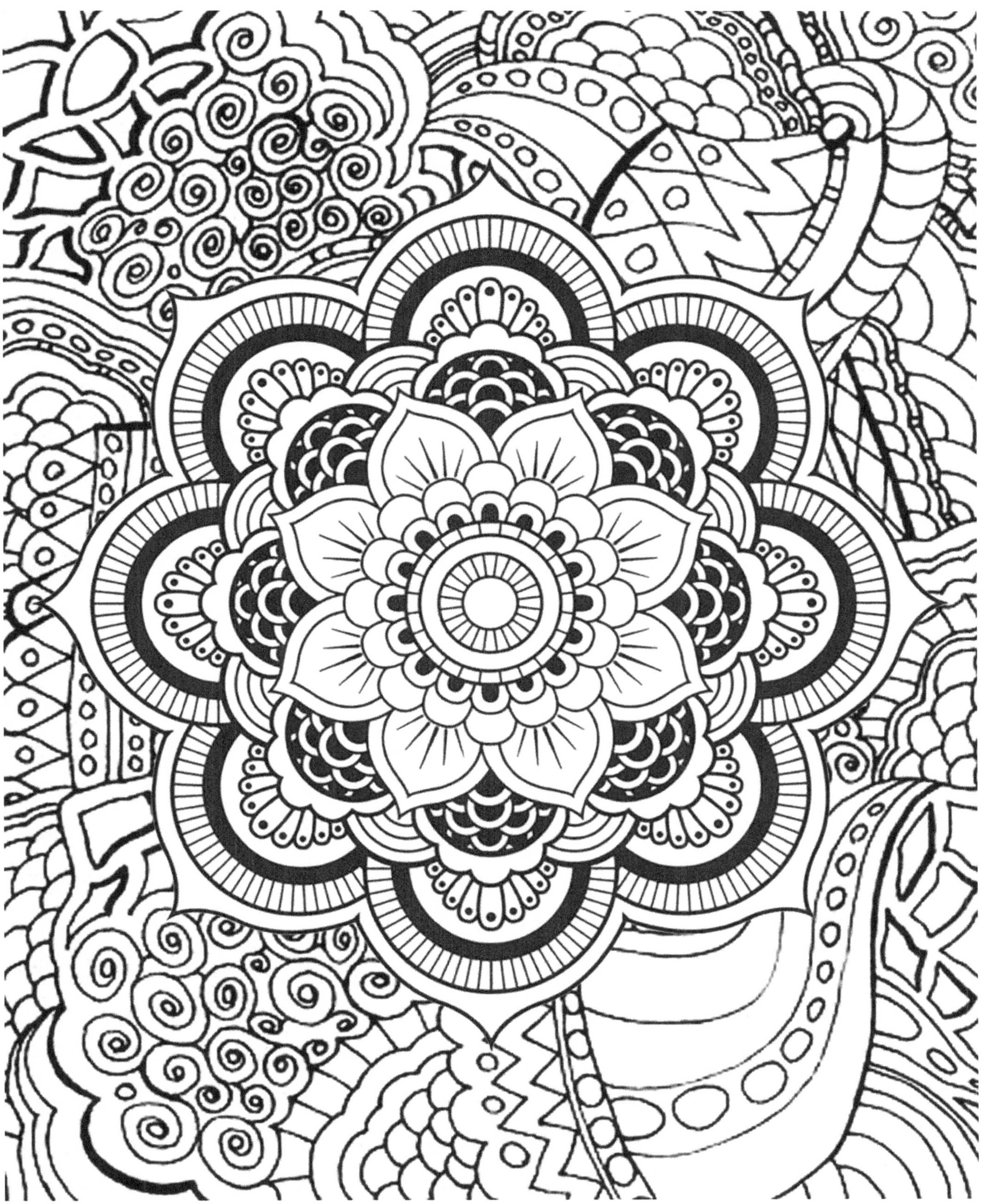

Lenka Sarkhelova

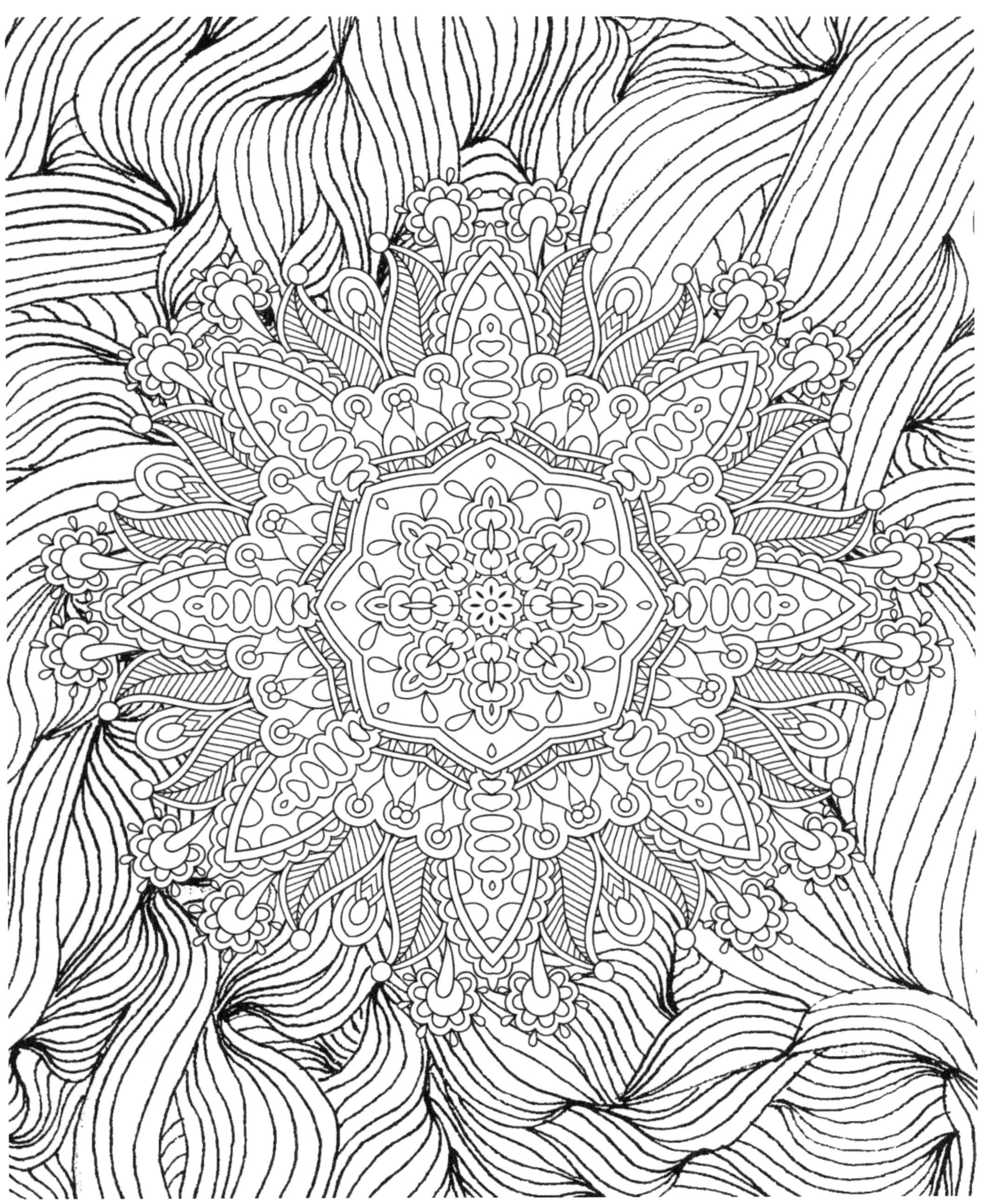

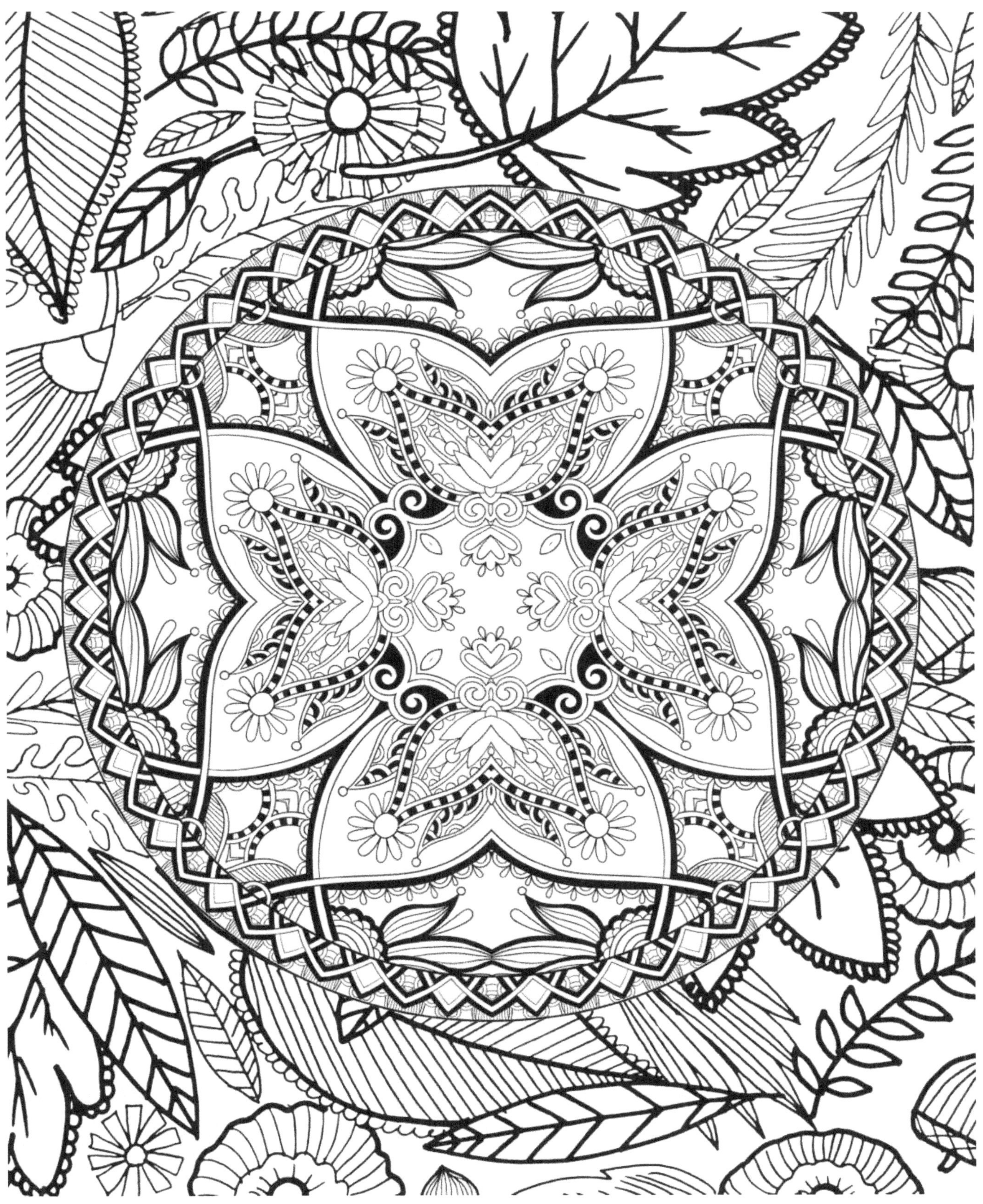

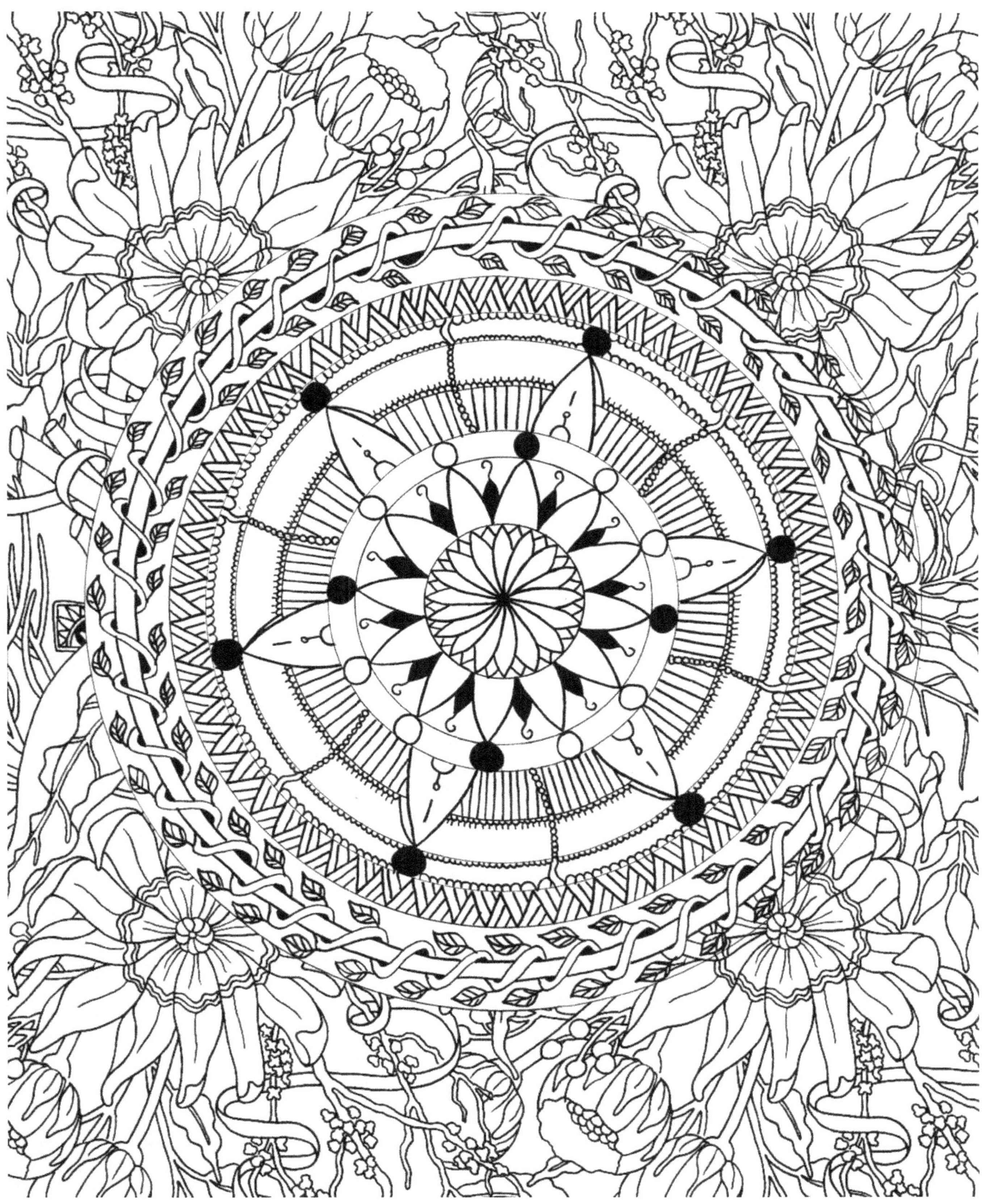

 

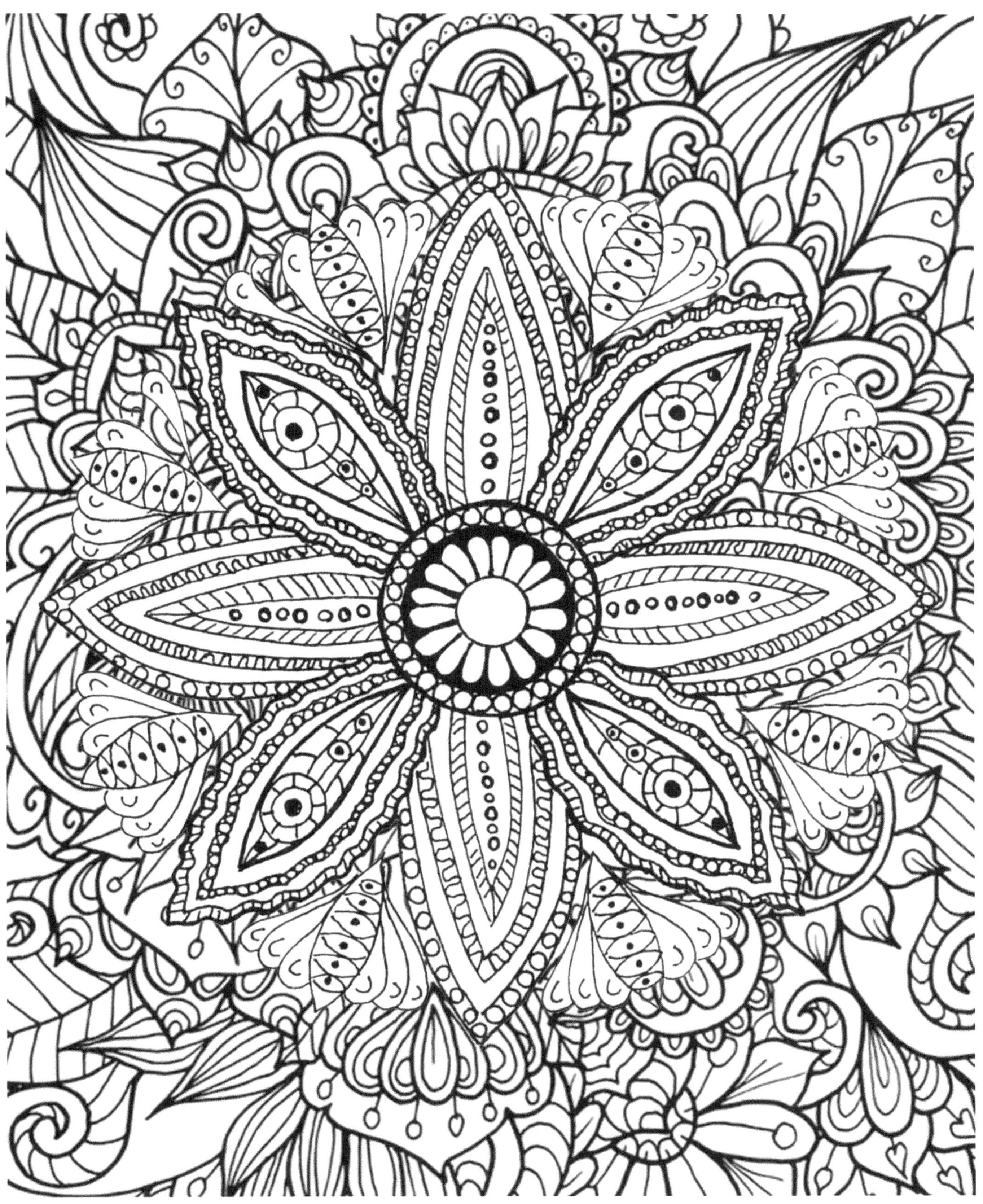

  

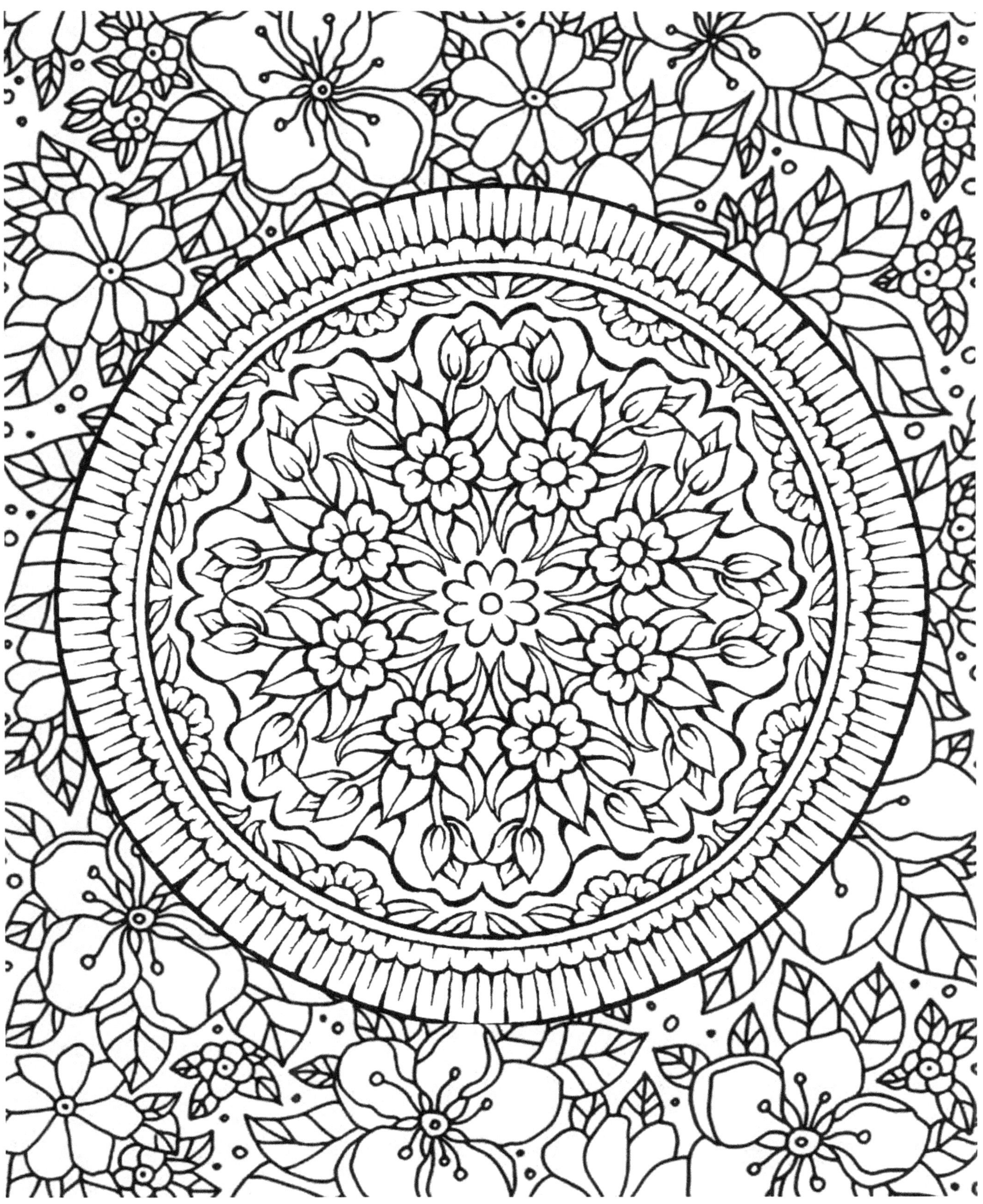

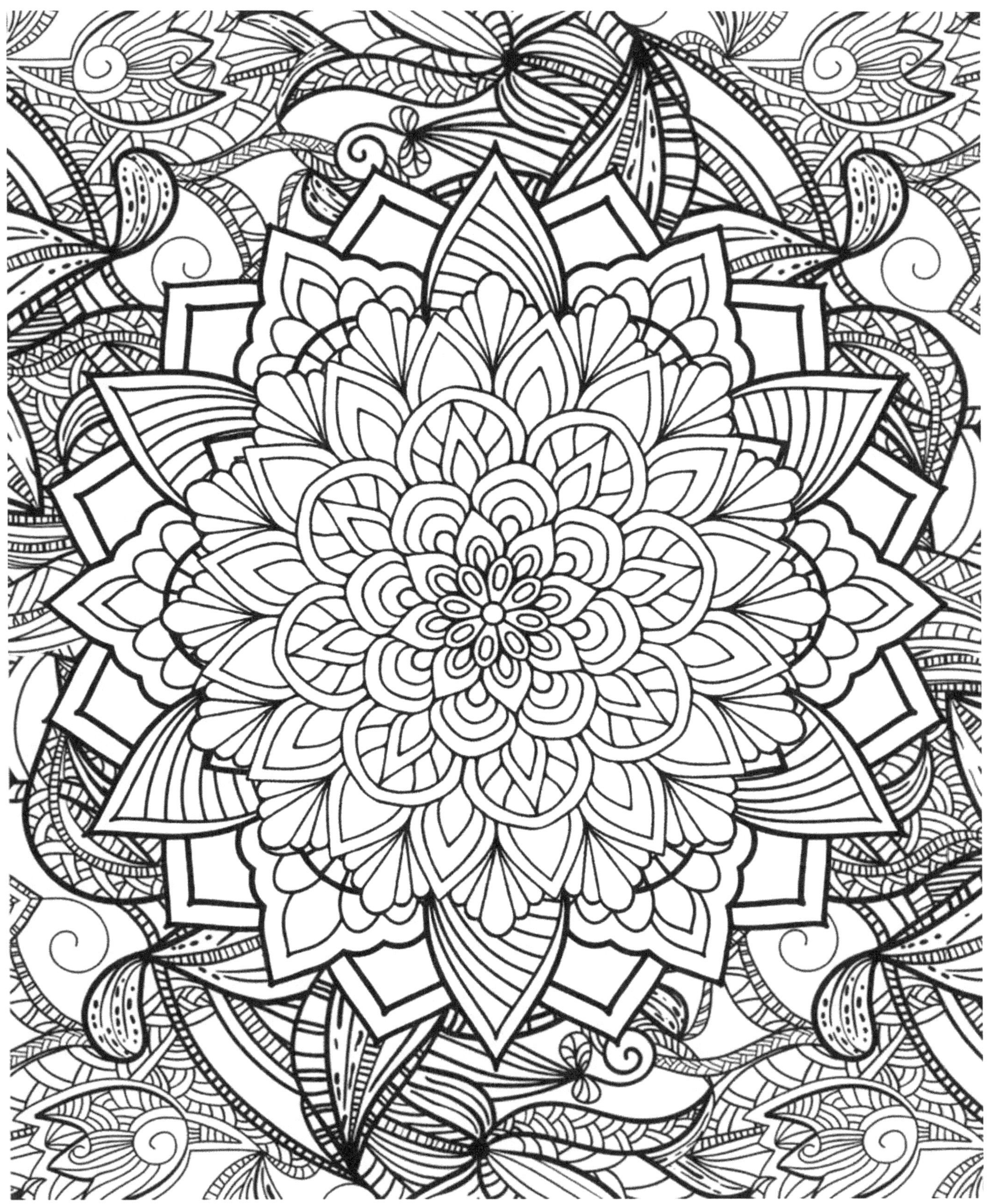

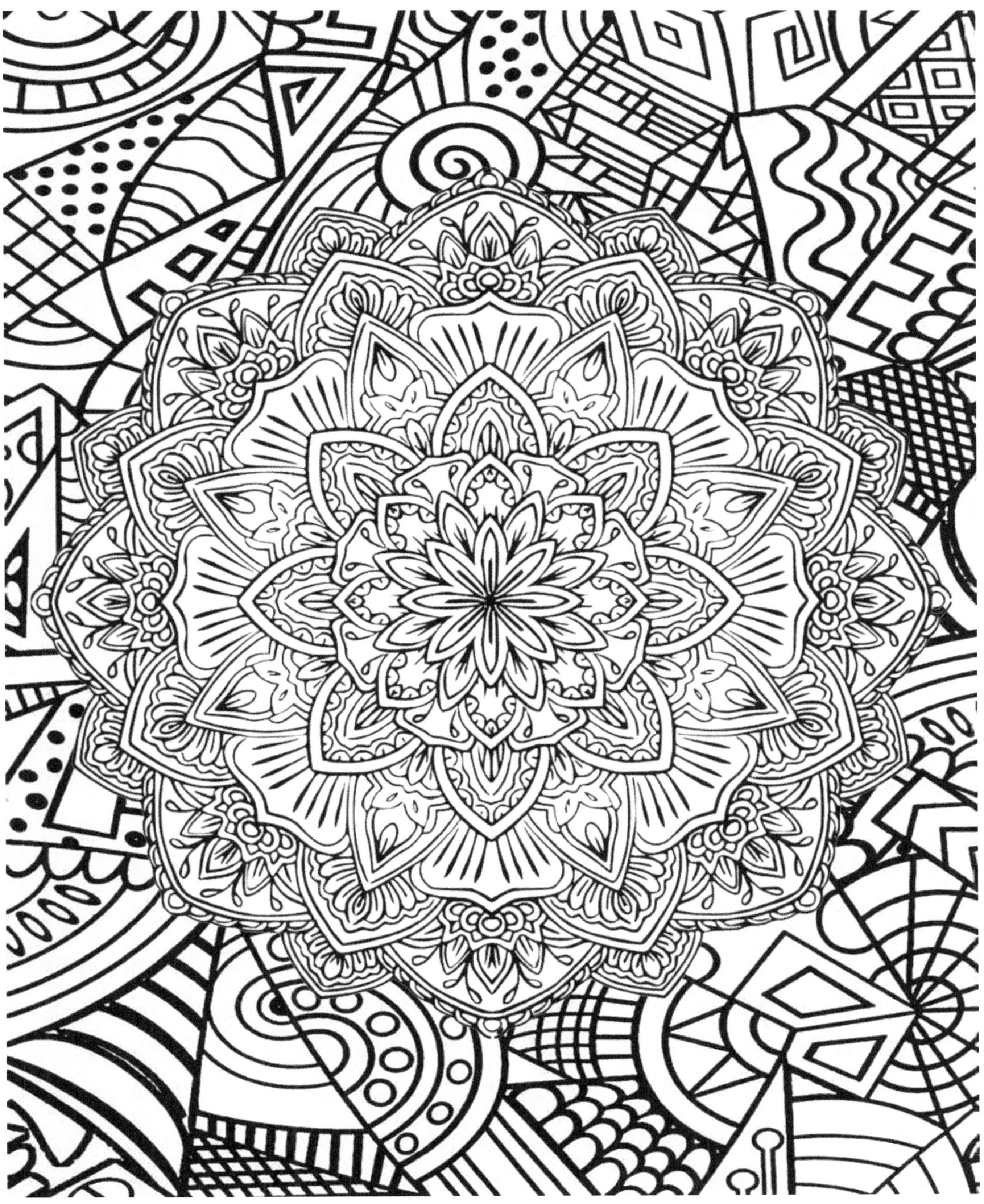

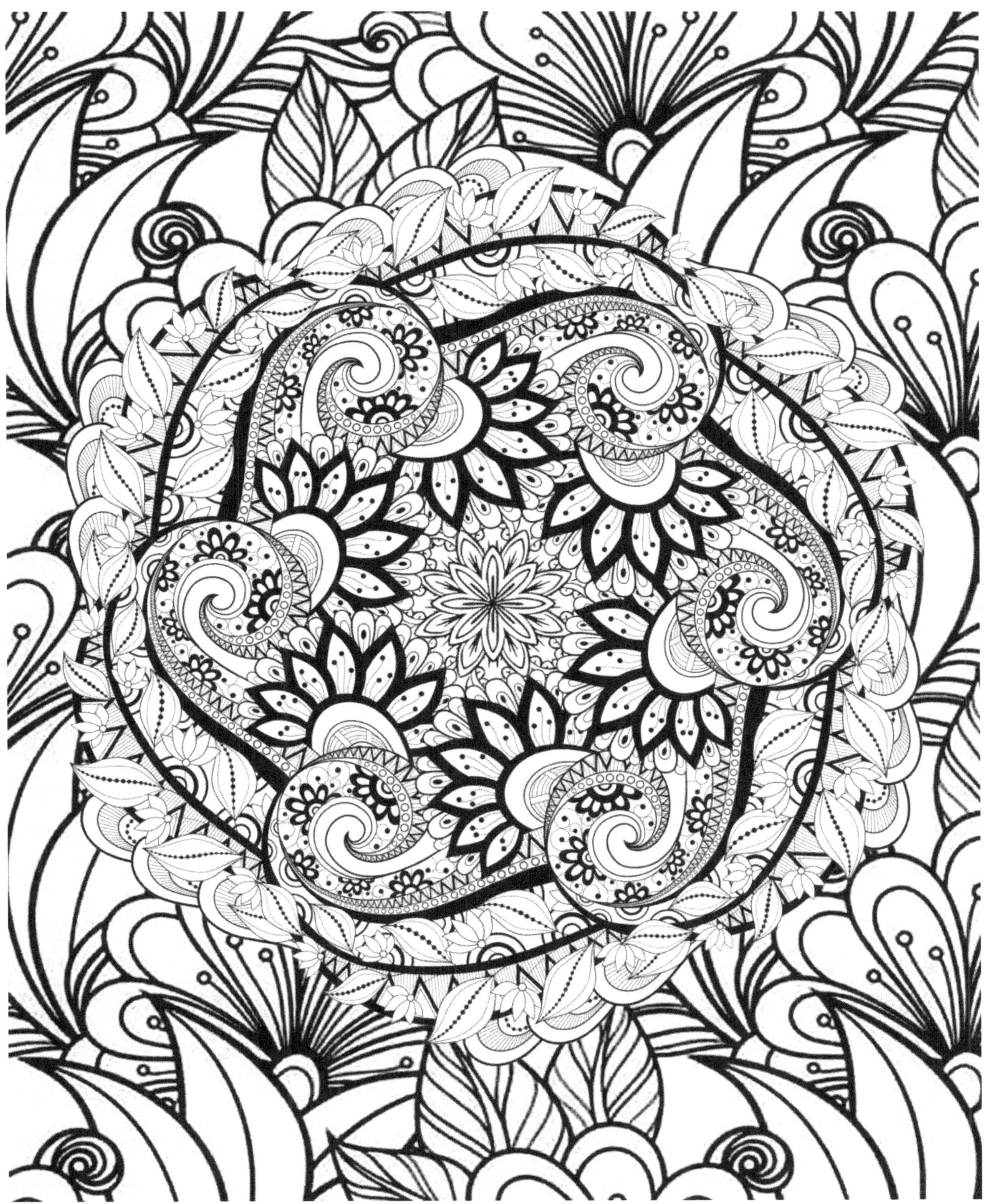

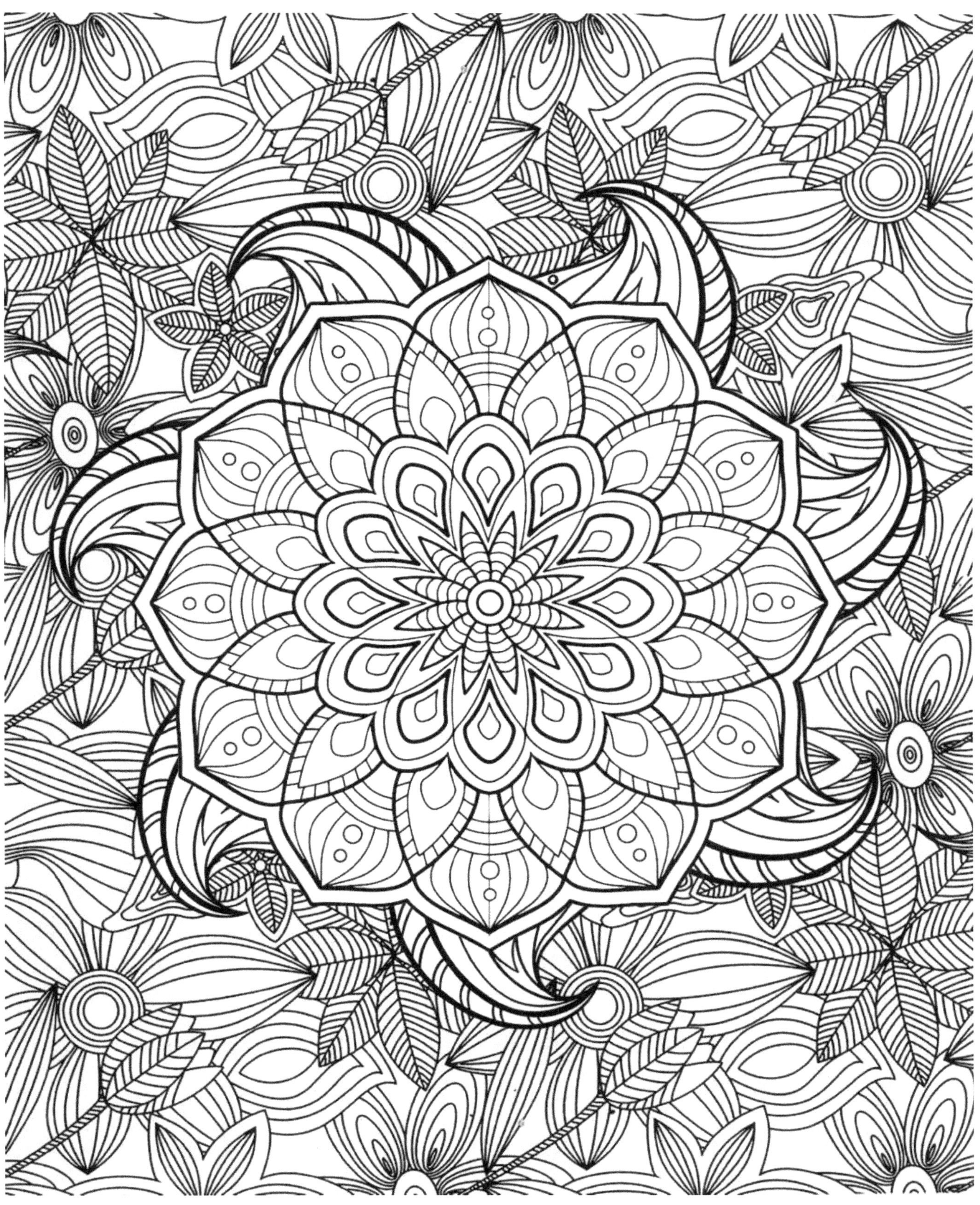

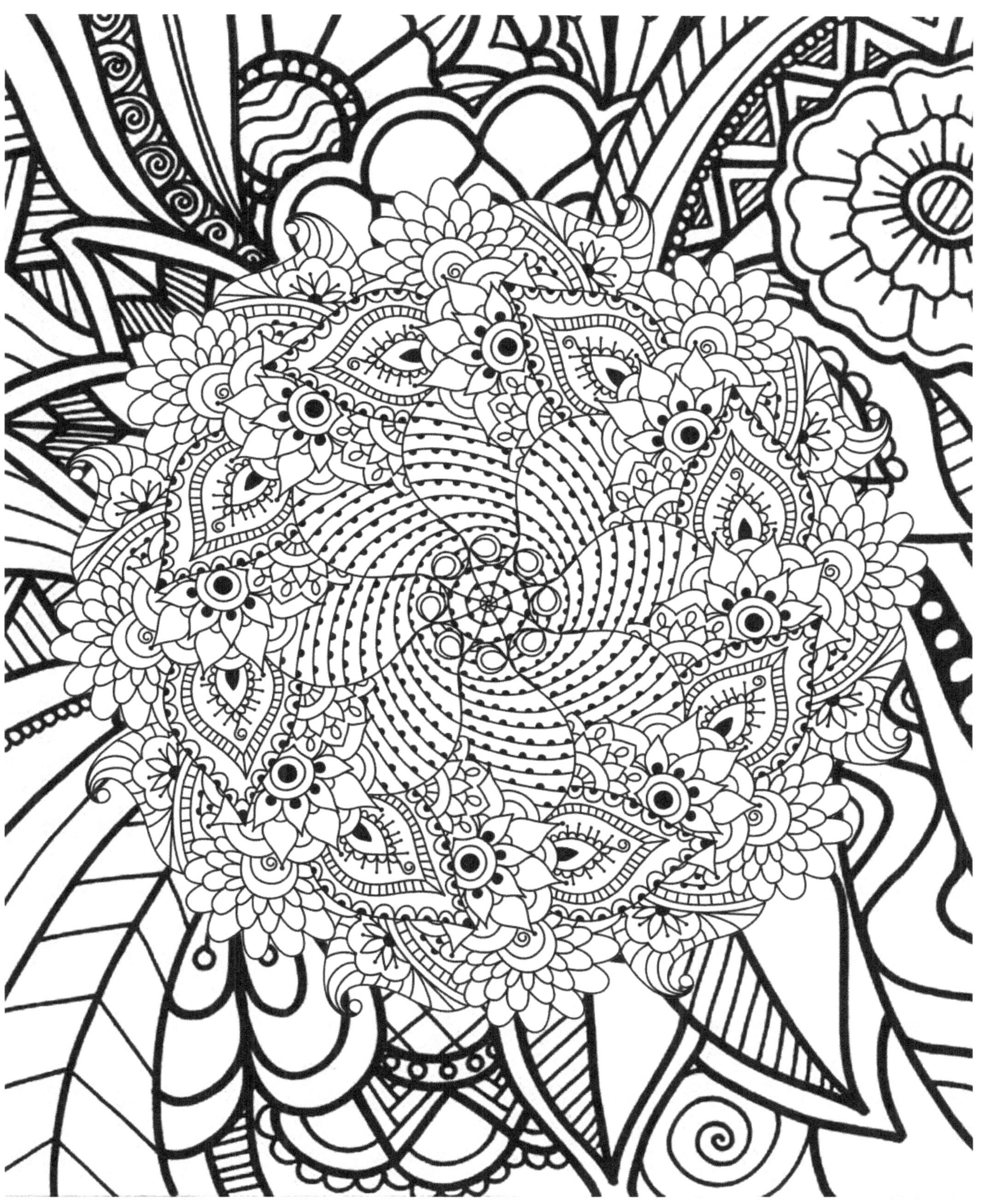

  Lenka Sarkhelova

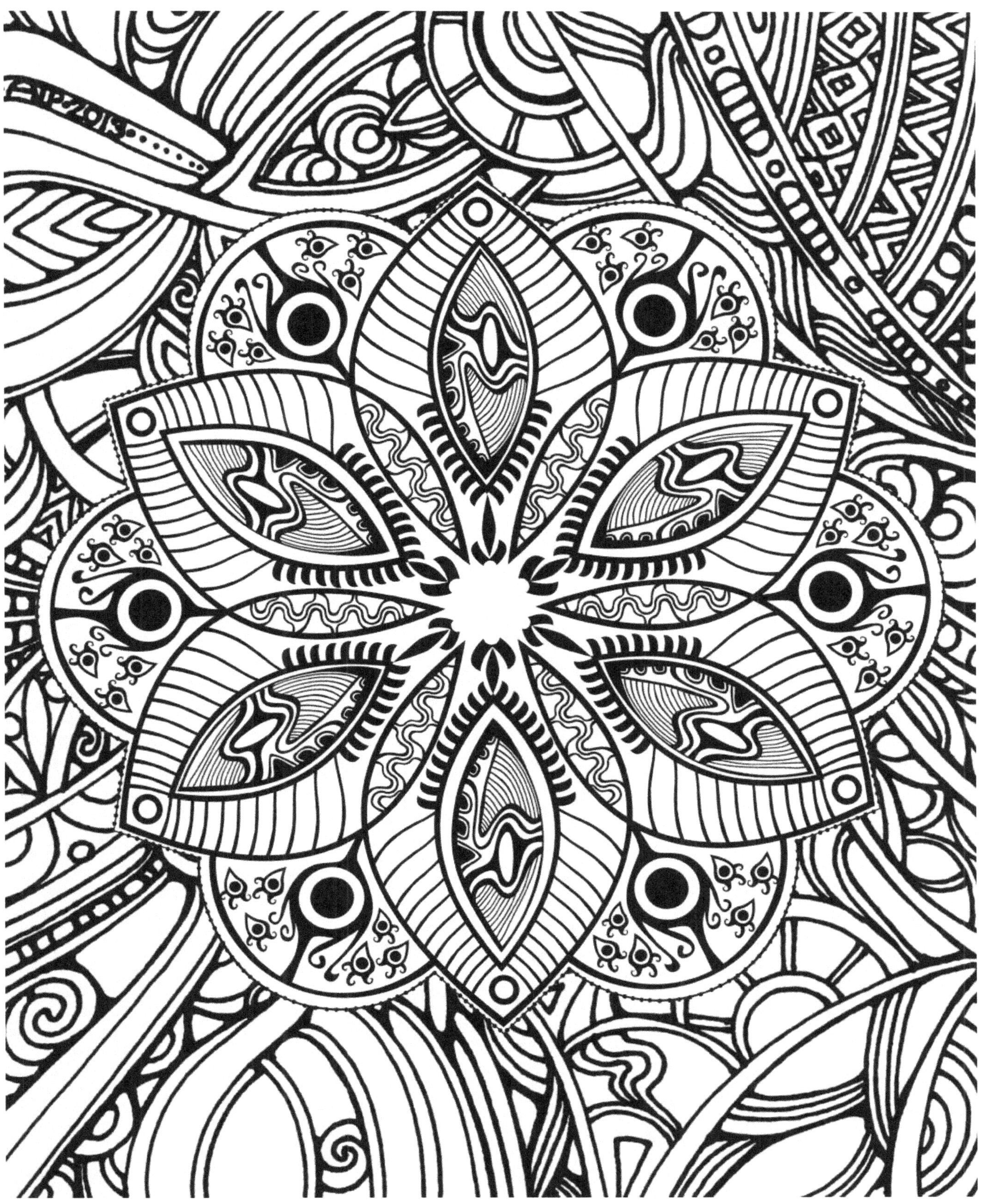

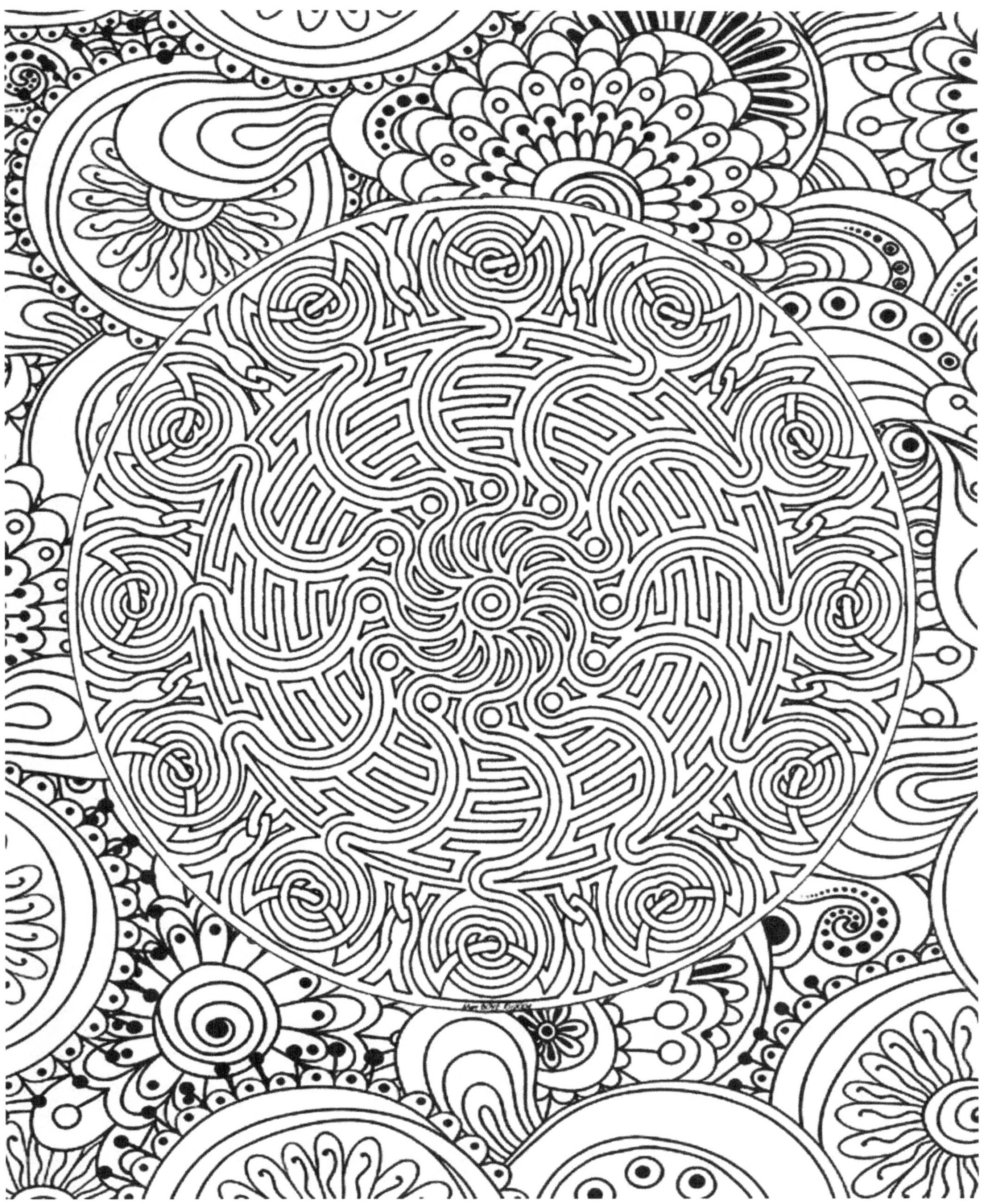

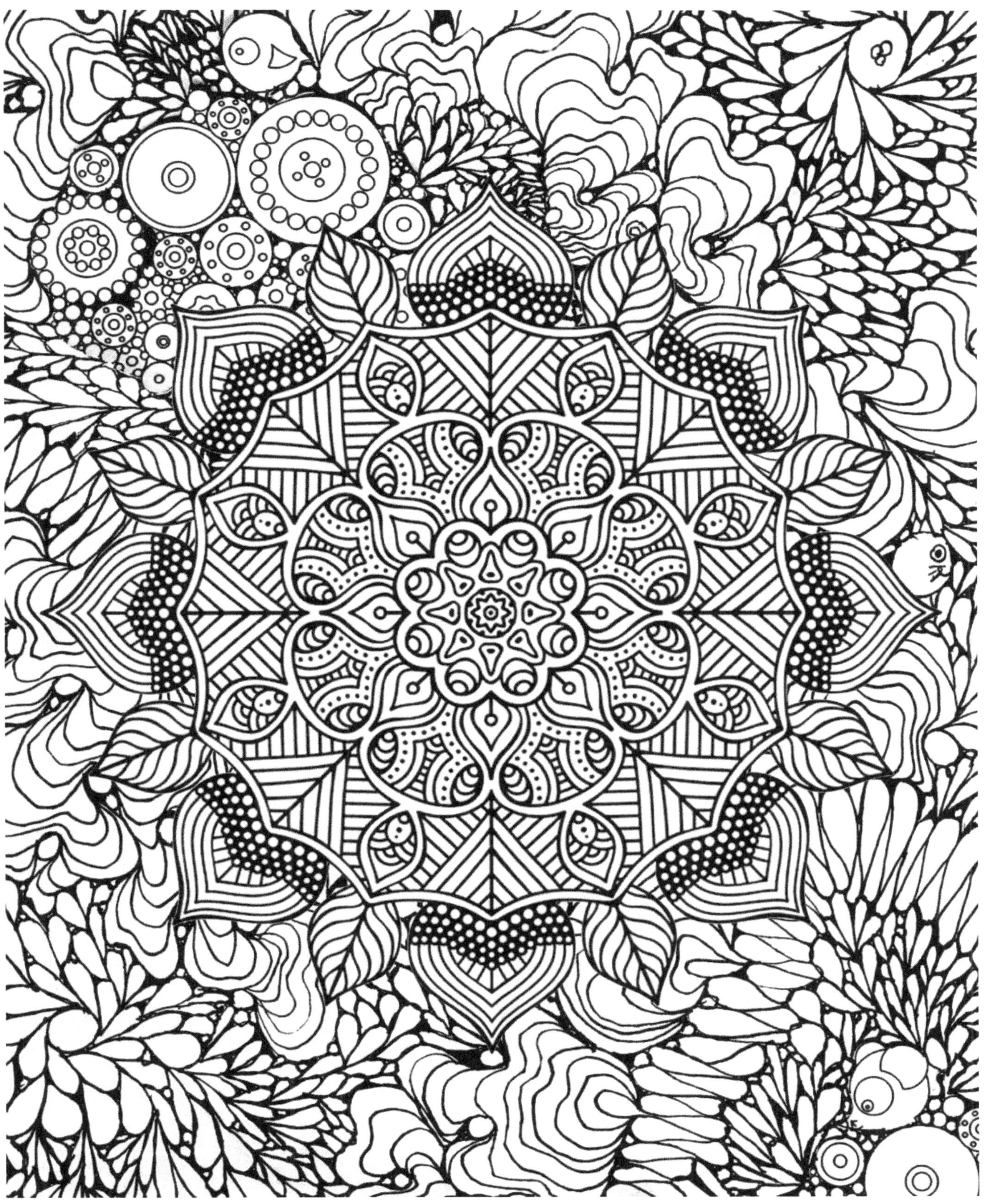

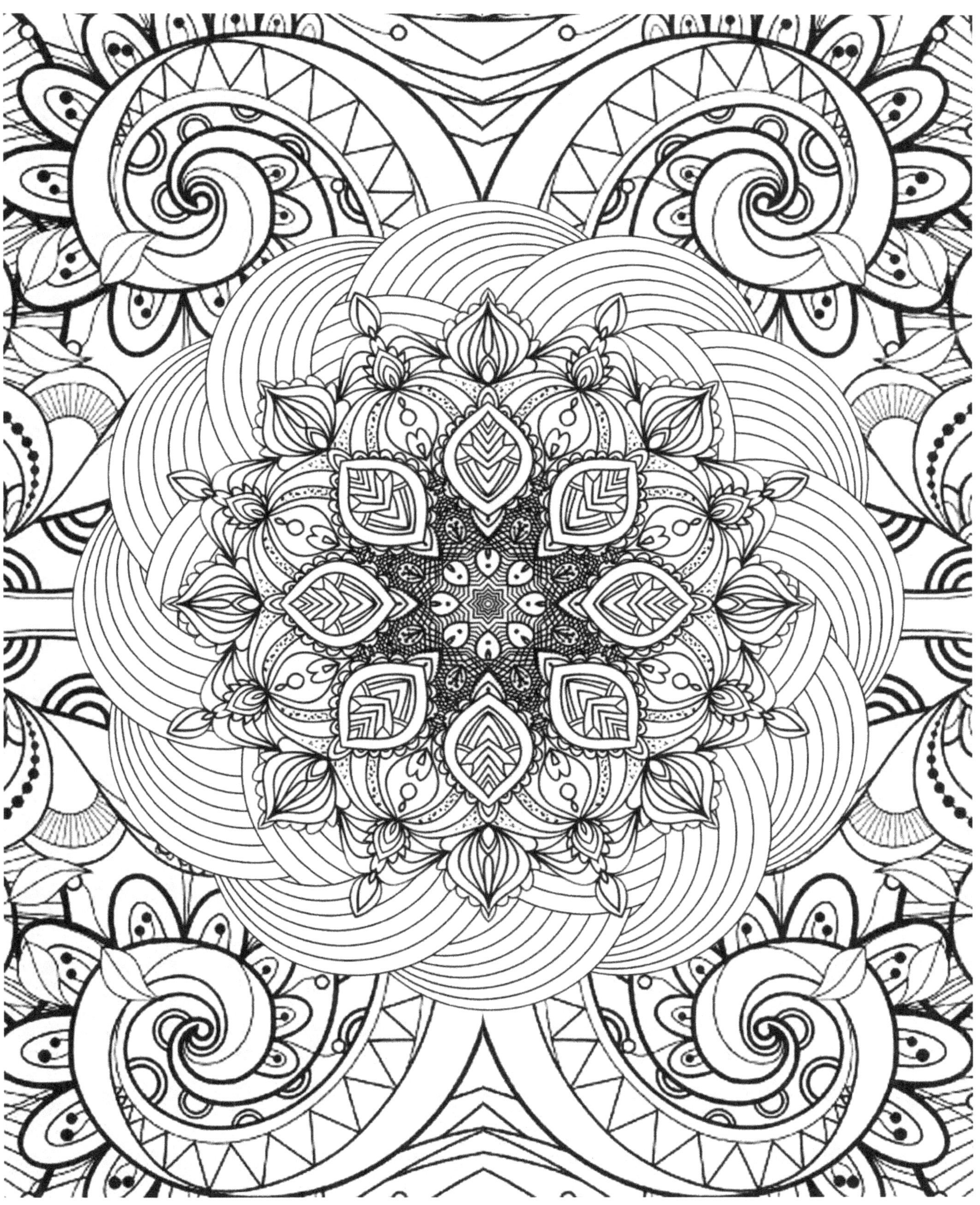

 

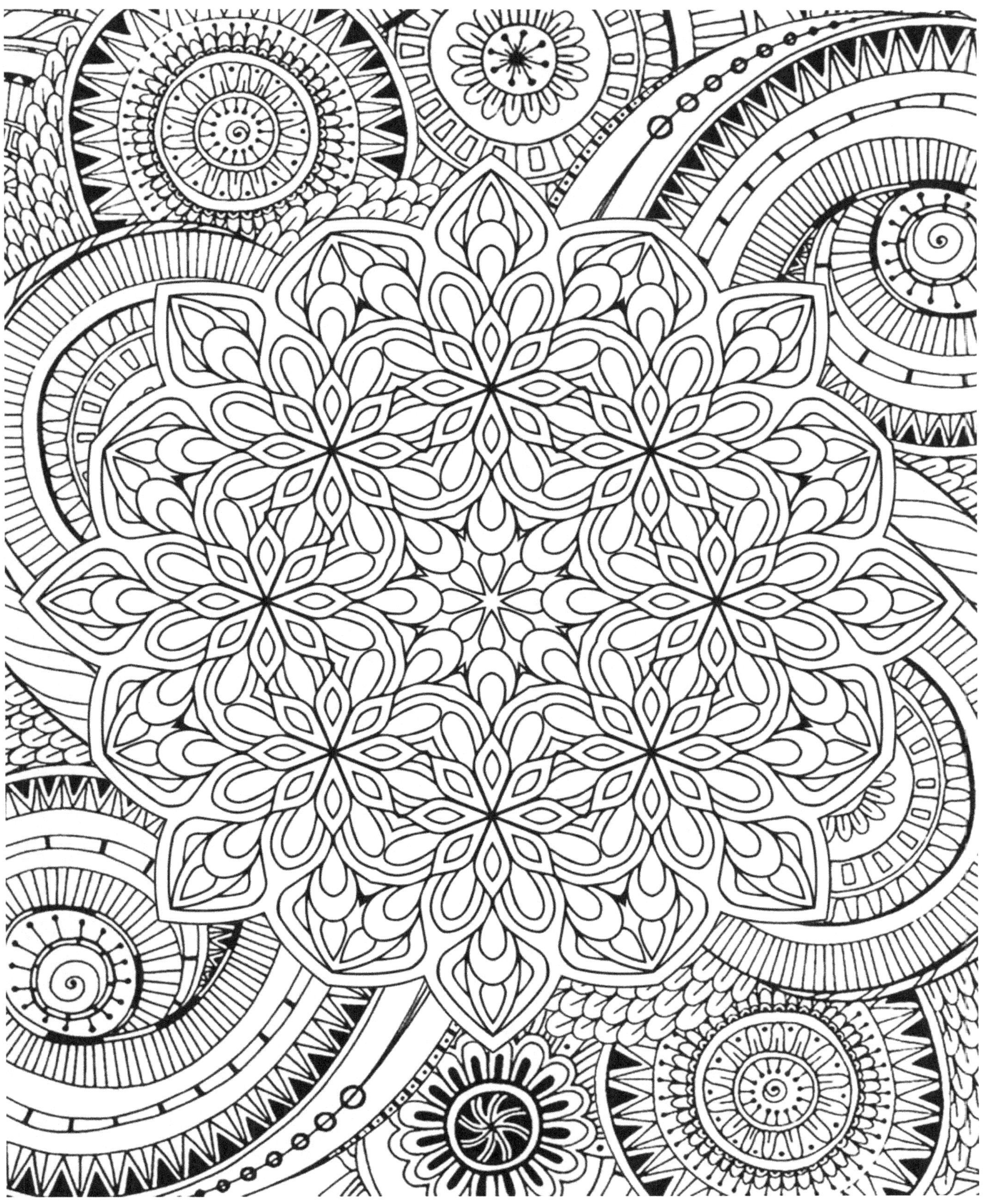

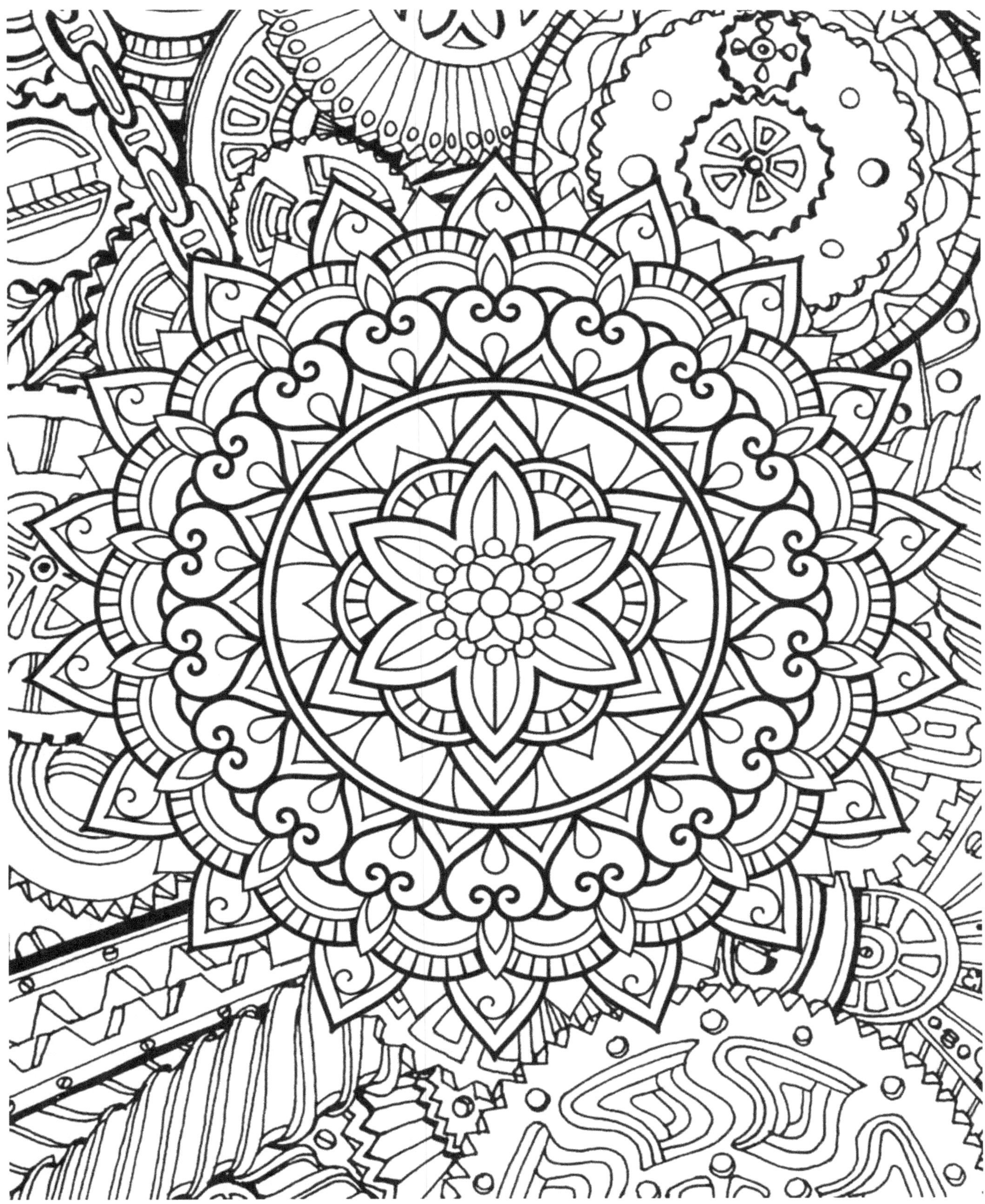

  

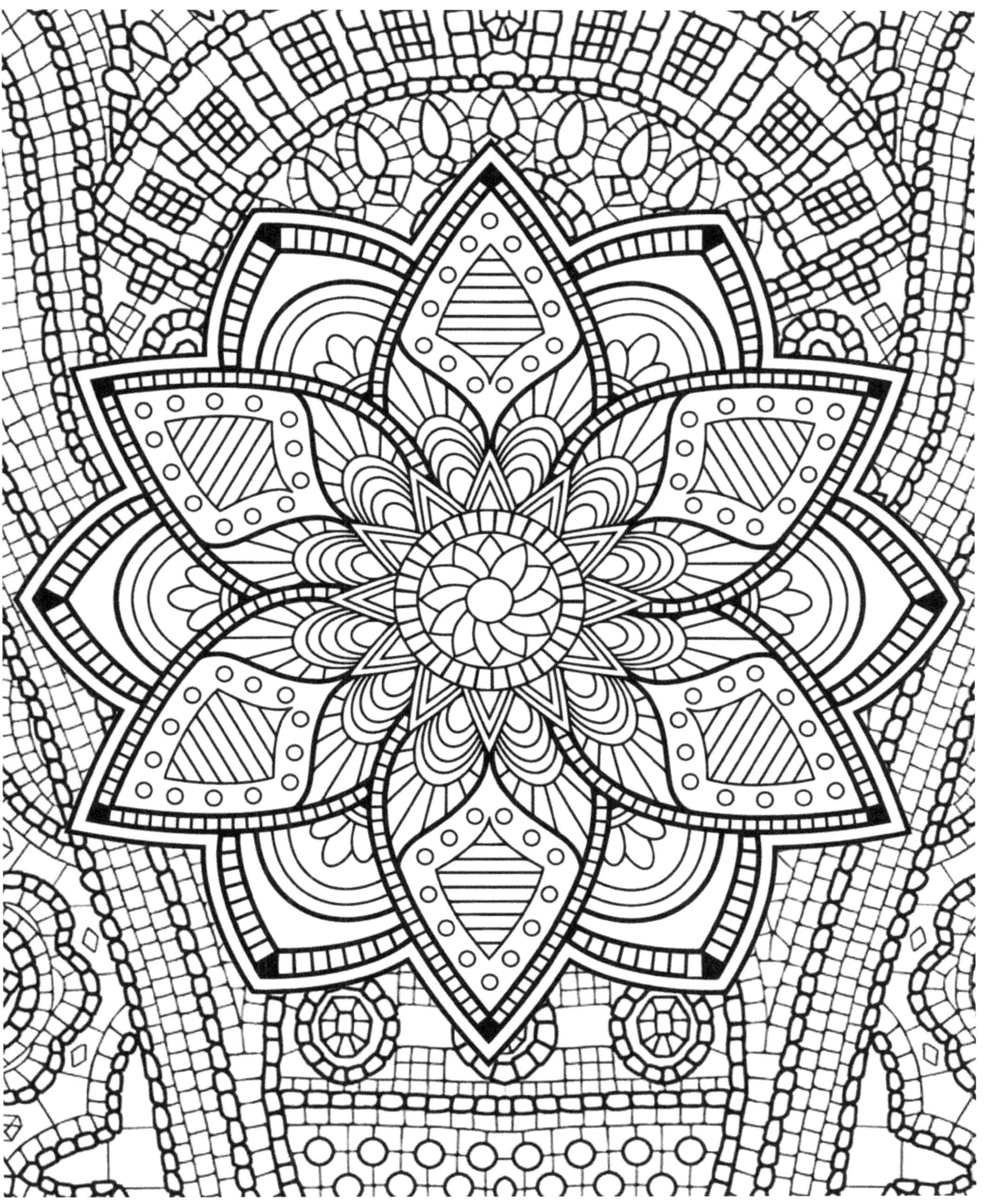

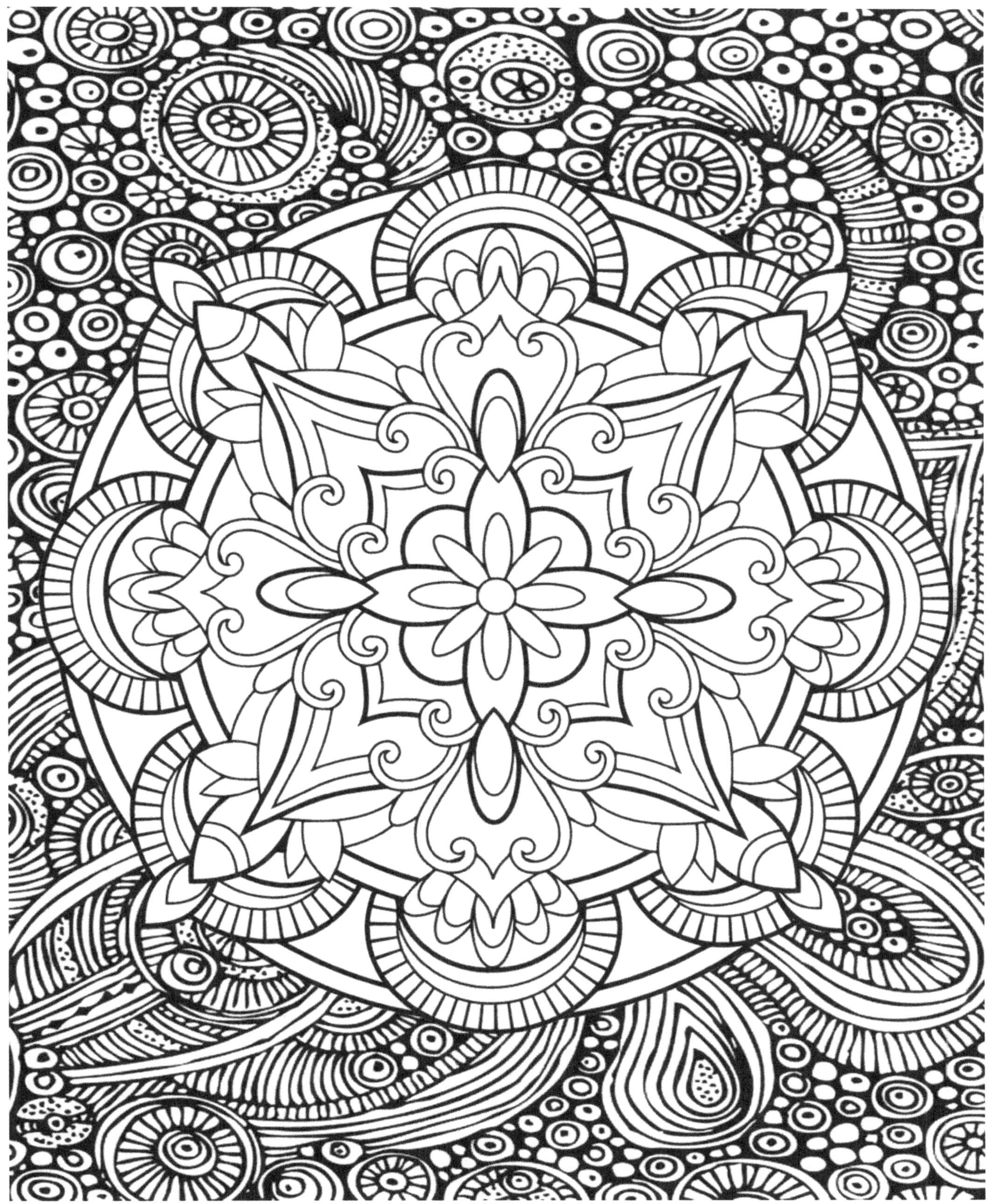

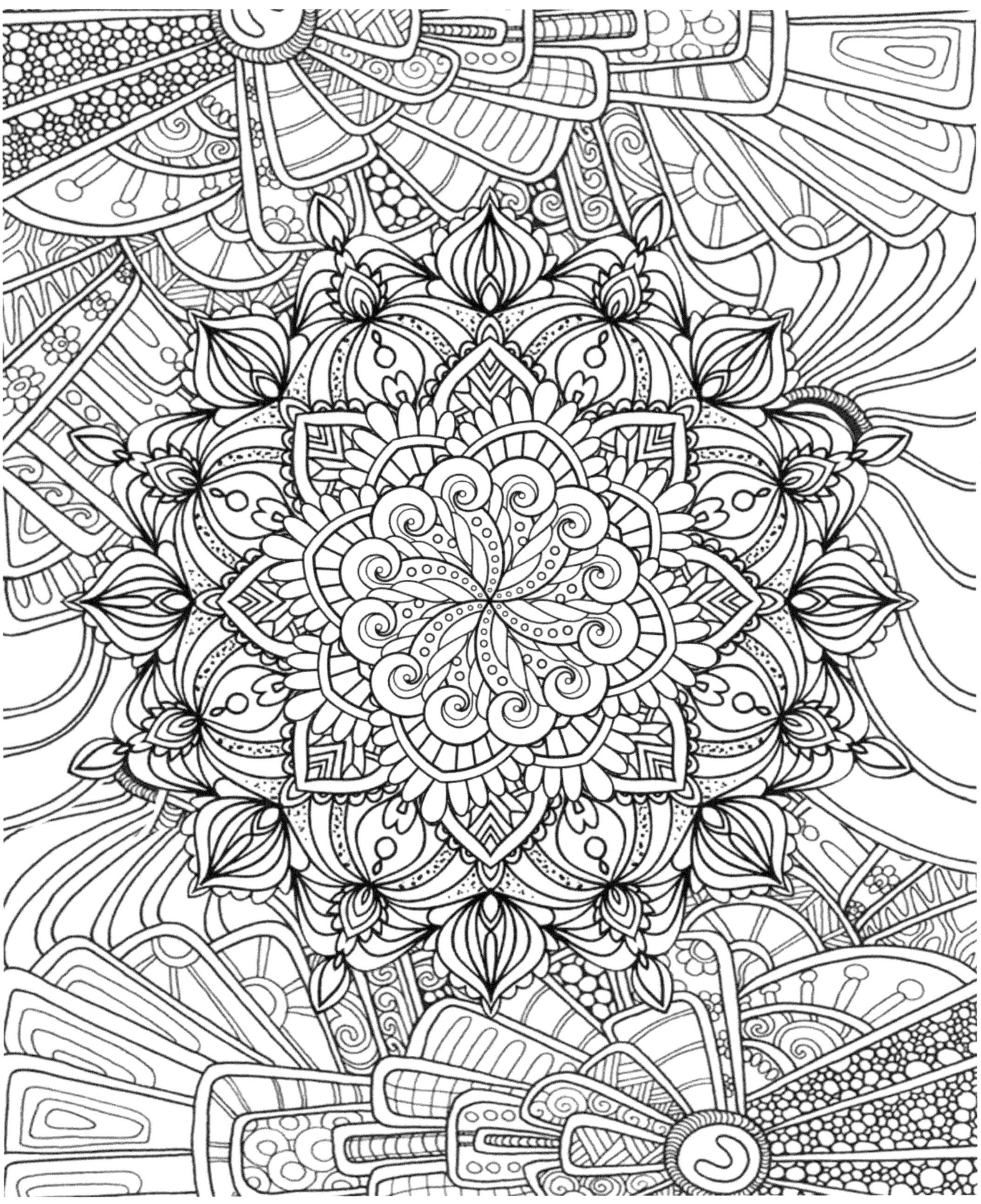

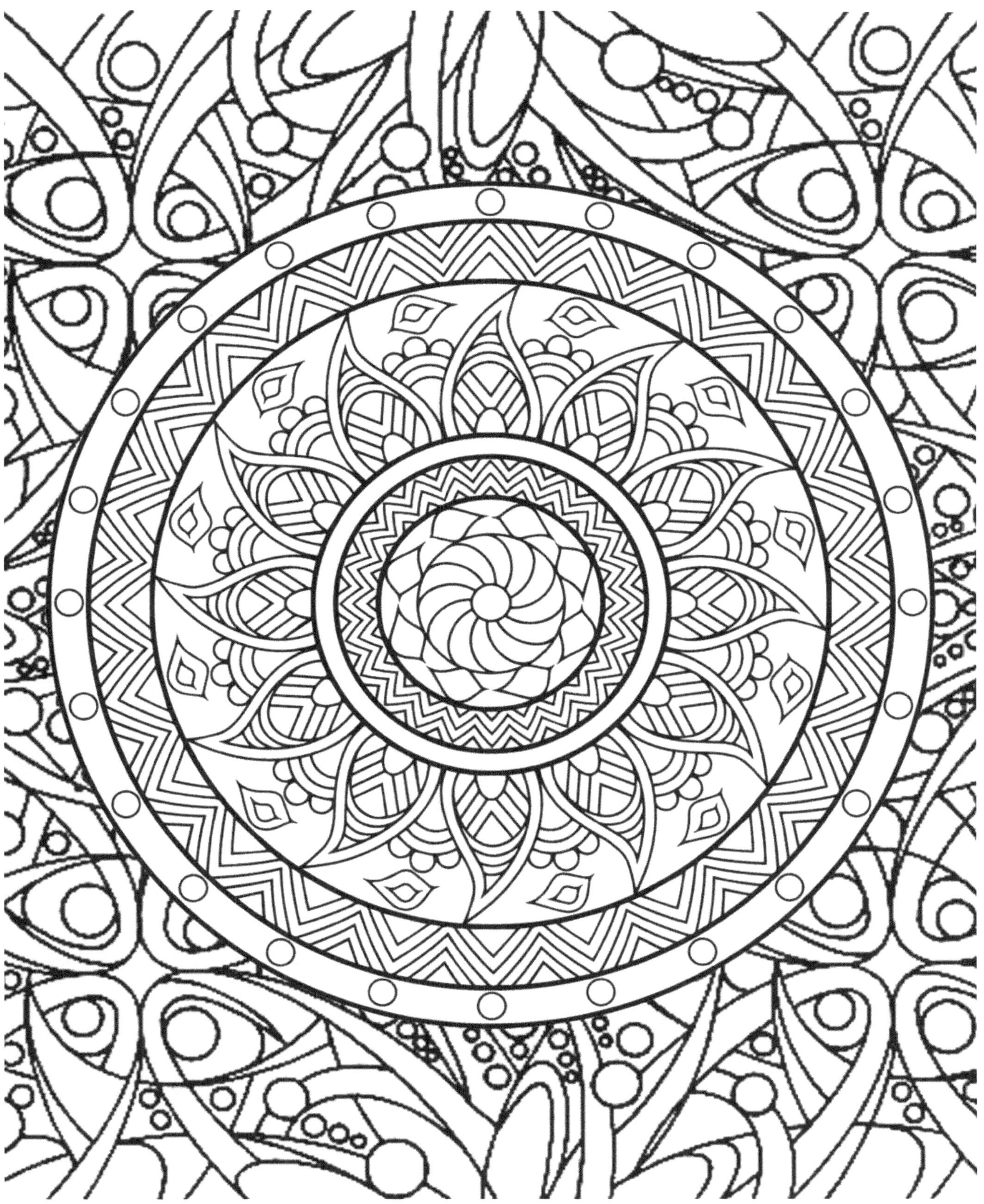